Vitamin C in Health and Disease

T. K. Basu, BVSc., MSc., PhD, Associate Professor of
Nutrition, University of Alberta, Edmonton, Canada

C. J. Schorah, BSc., PhD, Lecturer in Chemical Pathology,
University of Leeds, Leeds, England

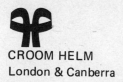

CROOM HELM
London & Canberra

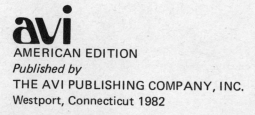

AMERICAN EDITION
Published by
THE AVI PUBLISHING COMPANY, INC.
Westport, Connecticut 1982

© 1982 T. K. Basu and C. J. Schorah
Croom Helm Ltd, 2–10 St John's Road, London SW11

British Library Cataloguing in Publication Data

Basu, T. K.
   Vitamin C in health and disease.
   1. Vitamin C metabolism
   I. Title   II. Schorah, C. J.
   613.2′8   QP772.A8

   ISBN 0-7099-0445-2

Published in North, Central and South America 1982 by
AVI PUBLISHING COMPANY, 250 Post Road East,
Westport, Connecticut 06881

ISBN 0-87055-406-9

Typeset by Pat Murphy, IBM Typesetting, 296b Lymington Road,
Highcliffe-on-Sea, Dorset, England.

Printed and Bound in Great Britain

CONTENTS

Foreword *Emil Ginter*

Acknowledgements

Introduction   9

1. Metabolism of Vitamin C   11
    1.1 Biosynthesis   11
    1.2 Absorption   13
    1.3 Tissue Distribution   15
    1.4 Turnover and Body Pool   16
    1.5 Catabolic Products and their Excretion   16
    1.6 Conclusions   20

2. The Estimation of Body Vitamin C Reserves   21
    2.1 Methods Available for the Assay of Vitamin C   21
    2.2 Preparation of the Sample   26
    2.3 Choice of Material for Assessment of Vitamin C
         Reserves   26

3. The Role of Vitamin C   38
    3.1 Vitamin C as a Reducing Agent   39
    3.2 Other Roles of Vitamin C   48
    3.3 Conclusions   58

4. Vitamin C Reserves and Requirements in Health and Disease   61
    4.1 Factors which Affect the Level of Plasma and
         Leucocyte Vitamin C in Health   64
    4.2 The Effect of Disease on Vitamin C Reserves   74
    4.3 Appropriate Vitamin C Reserves in Man   80

5. Therapeutic Aspects of Vitamin C   93
    5.1 Infectious Diseases   93
    5.2 Cardiovascular Disease   95
    5.3 Malignant Diseases   100
    5.4 Skeletal Disorders   107
    5.5 Tissue Healing   109
    5.6 Hypersensitivity   110

	5.7 Periodontal Disease	111
	5.8 Vitamin-sparing Effect	112
	5.9 Conclusions	113

6.	Safety Considerations on High Intake of Vitamin C	115
	6.1 Growth and Mortality Rate	115
	6.2 Protein and Amino Acid Metabolism	116
	6.3 Oxalate Excretion	117
	6.4 Gastrointestinal Disturbances	117
	6.5 Lysis of Erythrocytes	118
	6.6 Interaction with Warfarin	118
	6.7 Destruction of Vitamin B_{12}	119
	6.8 Bone Metabolism	119
	6.9 Infertility	120
	6.10 Adaptation to High Vitamin C Intake	121
	6.11 Effects on the Assay of Other Components in Biological Materials	121
	6.12 Conclusions	122

| 7. | General Conclusions | 124 |

| References | 128 |

| Index | 148 |

FOREWORD

The past decade has witnessed an information explosion on the subject of vitamin C, with some thousand new research papers appearing annually. Countless studies describe the role of vitamin C in the metabolism of connective tissue, particularly collagen, in cholesterol turnover, in immunological processes, in the detoxification of xenobiotics, in the transmission of interneuron information and in numerous other areas. Consequently, there is an urgent need that these facts be sorted out not only to facilitate their retrieval but also to promote an understanding of their significance for human health and disease alike.

Although an exact knowledge of the mechanisms involved in the biological functions of vitamin C still evades us today, new facts have helped us to realise that the need for vitamin C is not necessary uniquely for the prevention and treatment of scurvy. Classical medicine has failed to appreciate that scurvy is but the ultimate symptom of an absolute vitamin C deficiency and that there exists the danger of a covert marginal deficiency which is likely to disrupt the finer biochemical mechanisms and thereby bring about a deterioration of the health of large population groups. We are not as yet in a position to estimate precisely the degree of this risk to human health, but it is possible that a chronic vitamin C deficiency is involved in the origin of atherosclerosis and cancer — two of the biggest killers of mankind.

The authors of this monograph, Dr T. K. Basu and Dr C. J. Schorah, have eschewed the use of the simple method of uncritical compilation. Instead, they have focused particularly on the controversial problems. In many instances, the present state of knowledge does not permit them to draw definitive conclusions and, therefore, one should not look for many certainties in this domain. However what one will find here are intelligently asked questions. Although one need not and probably will not see eye to eye with everything presented by the authors (personally I consider the recommended daily dose of 60 mg vitamin C to be rather low), the book, as a whole, impresses the reader as being persuasive in its evidence, critical in its judgments and interpretations of data, restrained in its conclusions, but above all, as providing inspiration. Simultaneously, it provides a large quantity of well arranged documentary data on the metabolism of vitamin C and its biochemical rolcs, on the determination of body vitamin C reserves, on therapeutic aspects of ascorbic acid and on the risks possible in extreme vitamin C dosages.

As implied above, this book will not be the final word on the subject of biological roles of vitamin C, yet it will make readers think, whether they are vitaminologists, nutritionists, physicians, or one of the host of researchers concerned with problems relating to what we have come to call diseases of our civilisation.

Emil Ginter, PhD,
Institute of Nutrition,
Bratislava,
Czechoslovakia

ACKNOWLEDGEMENTS

The authors would like to thank colleagues, patients and volunteers whose contributions to, and assistance with, their work on vitamin C have helped to make this book possible. We would also like to thank our wives and families who have not only helped and encouraged us during the preparation of this book but who have also tolerated the disruption it has inevitably produced in family life.

INTRODUCTION

Scurvy, the deficiency disease which develops in the absence of adequate dietary vitamin C, was once a common condition in Europe but the introduction of root crops into the diet towards the end of the Middle Ages, unintentionally reduced the prevalence of the disease. Later the discovery that fruit juice could be used to treat sailors with scurvy (Lind, 1753) led eventually to the prevention of the disease during long sea voyages. The isolation of the antiscorbutic factor, vitamin C, from fruit juice (Szent-Györgi, 1928) would seem to complete the picture, all these factors helping to make a disease, common among the ancients, relatively rare in the United Kingdom today.

However, despite knowledge about its prevention, scurvy has not been eliminated and the incidence of the disease has recently been found to be surprisingly high in the elderly. In addition, although there has been considerable scientific investigation over the last 50 years, vitamin C itself remains an enigma. There are large differences in vitamin C reserves between different population groups, and recent evidence has suggested that in those groups where low levels are most frequently found, many individuals have reserves which are inappropriate. This situation is complicated by the fact that there is a difference of opinion on the amount of vitamin C to be recommended for daily ingestion, both in health and disease. Some workers hold the view that the requirement for this vitamin to maintain optimal health is much greater than is necessary for the prevention of scurvy. Furthermore, there is an increasing number of reports suggesting that the regular intake of vitamin C in large amounts is beneficial in a number of pathological conditions which are apparently quite unrelated to scurvy. Upon the existing evidence, it appears that these views are neither inadmissible nor incompatible. However, following publication of a popular book by Pauling (1970), there has been a widespread interest in self-medication with megadoses of vitamin C. This in turn has led to several clinical studies which have revealed little convincing evidence to support claims of clinical efficacy for megadose therapy, at least in most cases. Furthermore, in recent years there have been some isolated reports suggesting that the prolonged and regular intake of vitamin C in large doses may be potentially hazardous, at least to certain individuals.

All these claims certainly need to be evaluated.

The biochemical function of vitamin C is also unclear. Recent work has indicated a role for the vitamin in hydroxylation reactions. However, there is evidence for many other functions of vitamin C for which the mechanisms are not clearly understood.

It is these unresolved and often controversial areas that we have examined in most detail in this book. We have primarily considered evidence from research undertaken in the human, but have reported animal work where this has been appropriate. We have, in many cases, been unable to draw any final conclusions, but having critically summarised current evidence, we have made provisional recommendations, indicated those theories which seem the most probable, and suggested areas where further research is most needed. We have also suggested intakes and body reserves of vitamin C which, in the light of recent findings, should be appropriate for maintaining health and combating disease.

1 METABOLISM OF VITAMIN C

Vitamin C is essentially two compounds, L-ascorbic acid and its oxidised derivative L-dehydroascorbic acid. Although upwards of 90 per cent of vitamin C in animal tissues is in the form of ascorbic acid, both compounds have biological activity and are readily interconvertible by oxidation and reduction reactions through a short-lived intermediate, monodehydroascorbic acid (Equation 1.1). Some of the enzymes responsible for these interconversions are considered later (Section 3.1) and illustrated in Figure 3.1.

ascorbic acid   monodehydroascorbic acid   dehydroascorbic acid   (Eq. 1.1)

1.1 Biosynthesis

Most plants and animals have the ability to synthesise vitamin C from either D-glucose or D-galactose through the glucuronic acid pathway (Figure 1.1). There are, however, species which cannot synthesise the vitamin; in higher animals these are humans, guinea pigs, apes, fruit-eating bats and the red-vented bulbul (an Indian bird). In addition, there is evidence that insects, other invertebrates, fish and microorganisms are also incapable of synthesising vitamin C (Chatterjee *et al.*, 1975). These organisms lack enzymes in the biosynthetic pathway of the vitamin. Current evidence indicates that the defect in all vitamin C dependent species is the absence of the enzyme L-gulonolactone oxidase (Figure 1.1), which catalyses the final step in the biosynthesis of vitamin C (Burns, 1957; Sato, Nishikimi and Udenfriend, 1976; Sato and Udenfriend, 1978). A recent study has provided evidence showing that scurvy, the condition which develops in the absence of adequate tissue concentrations of vitamin C, can be prevented by providing this enzyme, together with its substrate L-gulonolactone, to guinea pigs (Sato, 1980). In practice, however, scurvy is prevented by providing

Figure 1.1: The Biosynthesis of L-Ascorbic Acid

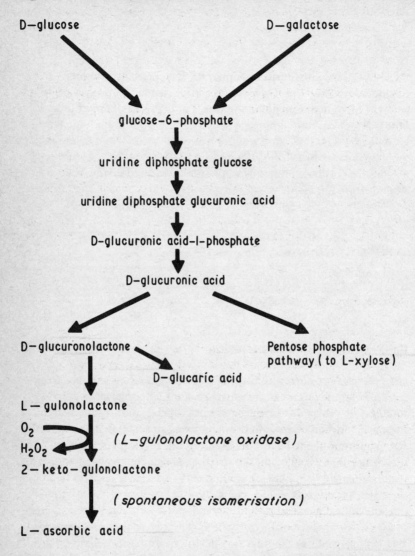

exogenous sources of vitamin C, and as a result this vitamin is considered to be an essential dietary requirement in the species lacking L-gulonolactone oxidase activity.

At the chromosomal level, the genes coding for the missing enzyme might be entirely absent as a consequence of deletion of genetic material (Burns, 1957). However, inability to demonstrate the biosynthesis of vitamin C in tissue homogenates does not necessarily signify absence of a particular enzyme. The defect could be due to the enzyme being deactivated by the products of the reaction. Thus it is possible that the formation of peroxide which accompanies the biosynthesis of 2-keto-gulonolactone (Figure 1.1) could be responsible for the deactivation of its parent enzyme, L-gulonolactone oxidase, in some species, thereby tending to inhibit this step in vitamin C biosynthesis.

Furthermore, the activity of L-gulonolactone oxidase may be subject to competitive inhibition with enzymes involved in the pentose phosphate (L-xylose) part of the biosynthetic fork (Lewin, 1976). In this context, it is noteworthy that vitamin C biosynthesis is known to occur in guinea pig embryos with rapidly differentiating tissues (De Fabro, 1967; Yew, 1975). It is possible that the competitive activities of the enzymes involved in the formation of L-xylose are less in the embryos than in the adults.

1.2 Absorption

In humans and guinea pigs, the absorption of vitamin C occurs in the buccal mucosa, stomach and small intestine (Figure 1.2). The uptake of vitamin C from solutions introduced into the buccal cavity of human subjects has been shown to be pH-dependent (Odumosu and Wilson, 1971). It also increases as the time of retention of the solution in the mouth is lengthened from one to five minutes. It is thought that the buccal absorption of vitamin C is mediated by passive diffusion through the membrane of the buccal mucosal cells. The rate and extent of diffusion are determined by the initial concentration of vitamin C in the buccal cells and by its rate of passage from the cells into the blood in the mucosal capillaries.

Gastrointestinal absorption of vitamin C in humans and guinea pigs has been found to be rapid and efficient, and an active carrier-mediated transport system has been put forward by many workers (Penney and Zilva, 1946; Stewart and Booth, 1964; Kubler and Gehler, 1970; Mayersohn, 1972). However, in species with no dietary requirement for vitamin C, such as rats and hamsters, the mode of intestinal absorption of the vitamin has been demonstrated to be passive transport (Spencer *et al.*, 1963).

Using perfused intestinal segments, Stevenson and Brush (1969)

Figure 1.2: The Absorption and Distribution of Vitamin C

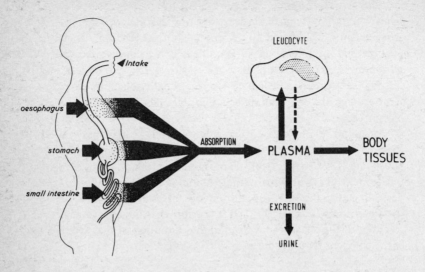

studied vitamin C absorption in the guinea pig. The results of this study
have revealed that the vitamin is absorbed from the distal region of the
small intestine of the guinea pig by an active transport system which
has the characteristics of a sodium-dependent coupled-carrier
mechanism. These workers postulated that the mode of intestinal
transport for a given species would reflect the presence or absence of a
dietary requirement for vitamin C. Thus in species such as the guinea
pig, the vitamin would be absorbed by active transport, and in the
species that produce vitamin C endogenously, such as the rat, the
absorption would occur passively.

In man, the sodium-dependent active transport mechanism appears
to occur at low concentrations of vitamin C (Tolbert *et al.*, 1967).
However, this active absorption mechanism becomes saturated when the
mucosal concentration of the vitamin is greater than 6 millimolar. This
may account for the fact that the proportion of dietary vitamin C
absorbed decreases with increasing intake of the vitamin (Hornig,
Vulleumier and Hartmann, 1980).

It is thought that the absorption of vitamin C is facilitated by
conversion to its oxidised form, dehydroascorbate. This may be due to
the fact that unlike vitamin C, the dehydroascorbate, which is less
ionised at physiological pH, has marked mebrane-penetrating power. It

is of further interest that the rate of transfer of dehydroascorbate into the blood is very low and once it has entered the gastrointestinal epithelium it appears to be rapidly reduced within the cell to ascorbic acid.

1.3 Tissue Distribution

Transfer of vitamin C occurs between plasma and leucocytes, and plasma and other tissues (Figure 1.2). The lowest concentrations of vitamin C appear to be in the plasma (Table 1.1). This indicates that transfer of the vitamin from blood to tissue must occur against a concentration gradient and therefore to be mediated through active

Table 1.1: Vitamin C Content of Adult Human Tissues

Tissue	Vitamin C (mg/100 g wet tissue)
Pituitary gland	40−50
Adrenal glands	30−40
Eye lens	25−31
Brain	13−15
Liver	10−16
Spleen	10−15
Kidneys	5−15
Heart muscle	5−15
Lungs	7
Skeletal muscle	3
Testes	3
Thyroid	2
Leucocytes	35
Plasma	0.4−1.0

transport mechanisms. Although no particular organ acts as a storage reservoir for the vitamin, the tissues, and leucocytes in particular, must be regarded as a storehouse for it. This may account for the fact that scurvy only becomes clinically apparent after a subject has been on a vitamin C free diet for several weeks.

It is not the dietary intake of vitamin C alone which determines tissue saturation. Several other factors are known to have an influence on vitamin C storage (Wilson, 1977). These include: metabolic factors which are associated with low vitamin C levels in particular tissues; patho-physiological factors which may give rise to acute and continuing tissue desaturation of the vitamin while the factors continue to operate; and iatrogenic factors which continue to operate while the causative drug is being administered. All these factors may increase the tissue demand of the vitamin and as a consequence may result in a degree of tissue desaturation which will be relative to one's vitamin C status to begin with (Chapter 4).

1.4 Turnover and Body Pool

The average half-life of vitamin C in an adult human is about 16 days, with a turnover of 1 mg/kg/day and a body pool of 22 mg/kg (Hellman and Burns, 1958). More recently, Baker, Saari and Tolbert confirmed that in healthy men with a dietary intake of about 100 mg vitamin C daily, the half-life of vitamin C is about 20 days and the body pool 2—3 g. The pool size may also be related to the fat-free body weight and was found to be 32—34 mg/kg fat-free mass in five men (Baker, Saari and Tolbert, 1966).

Using labelled vitamin C, Baker and his associates (1971) performed metabolic studies in five healthy adult male volunteers during both depletion and repletion of the vitamin. This study revealed that there was a direct relationship between clinical signs of scurvy and the pool size of vitamin C. Frank signs of scurvy were observed in all subjects when the body pool of the vitamin had been depleted to a level of 300 mg, and the clinical signs began to disappear when repletion took the vitamin C pool above a level of 300 mg.

More recent studies involving healthy male volunteers have demonstrated that the half-life of vitamin C is inversely related to its dosage and that the pool could be increased by increasing the dosage (Kallner, Hartmann and Hornig, 1977, 1979). It also appears from these studies that the saturated pool size could be reached by a daily intake of about 100 mg vitamin C in 95 per cent of the healthy population.

1.5 Catabolic Products and their Excretion

Using $(1-^{14}C)$-ascorbic acid, it has been shown that in guinea pigs about 60—70 per cent and in rats about 20—30 per cent of the vitamin ingested, is converted to CO_2 and excreted in the breath (Hornig, 1975).

Similar studies in human subjects, however, have revealed that the respiratory route is not a major pathway for vitamin C elimination (Hellman and Burns, 1958; Baker *et al.*, 1969, 1971). Thus less than 2 per cent of the ingested $(1-^{14}C)$-ascorbic acid has been shown to be excreted by exhalation in humans. It appears, therefore, that there is a fundamental difference in the elimination of vitamin C in humans from that of rats and guinea pigs.

In addition to CO_2, vitamin C may be oxidised to a variety of products in both humans and animals. Vitamin C is first oxidised to monodehydroascorbate, a free radical intermediate which exists in a very small concentration but has been detected by electron spin resonance (Equation 1.1). This metabolite is then further oxidised to dehydroascorbate, a stable lactone, which is hydrolysed to a relatively unstable intermediate, 2,3-diketogulonic acid. Subsequently, this compound decomposes to a variety of products as shown in Figure 1.3.

Perhaps the best known of these metabolites of vitamin C to be found in the urine is oxalic acid, which is derived from the 1- and 2- carbons of the vitamin by C_2-C_3 cleavage (Figure 1.3). Although this metabolite accounts for only 5–10 per cent of the excretion products of vitamin C, it seems to be an essential metabolite since it has been found to be present in urine even in the face of severe depletion of the vitamin C pool in humans (Baker *et al.*, 1971). Excretion of vitamin C in man can therefore occur in the form of the vitamin itself (ascorbic acid) and diketogulonate, L-xylose, traces of CO_2 and oxalate (Baker, Saari and Tolbert, 1966; Baker, 1967).

Another metabolite of vitamin C found to be present in both human and guinea pig urine is ascorbic acid-2-sulphate (Baker *et al.*, 1971). It has been suggested that the presence of this sulphated derivative in urine is only easily observed on a restricted vitamin C intake, since excretion of unchanged vitamin C normally masks its presence. Ascorbate-2-sulphate has been considered to be a vitamin in fish, but it does not seem to prevent scurvy in guinea pigs or monkeys (Kuenzig, Avenia and Kamm, 1974).

The demonstration of ascorbate-2-sulphate in human urine as well as in the urine of guinea pigs, suggests that this compound is a common metabolite of vitamin C, but the question of whether it is an active metabolite or simply a metabolic end product has not yet been determined. However, a number of biological roles for this sulphated derivative of vitamin C have been suggested. It could act as a sulphate donor as suggested by Chu and Slaunwhite (1968). It also seems possible that ascorbate-2-sulphate plays a role in the transfer of

Figure 1.3: The Vitamin C Complex and its Degradation Products. The complete process is not fully established.

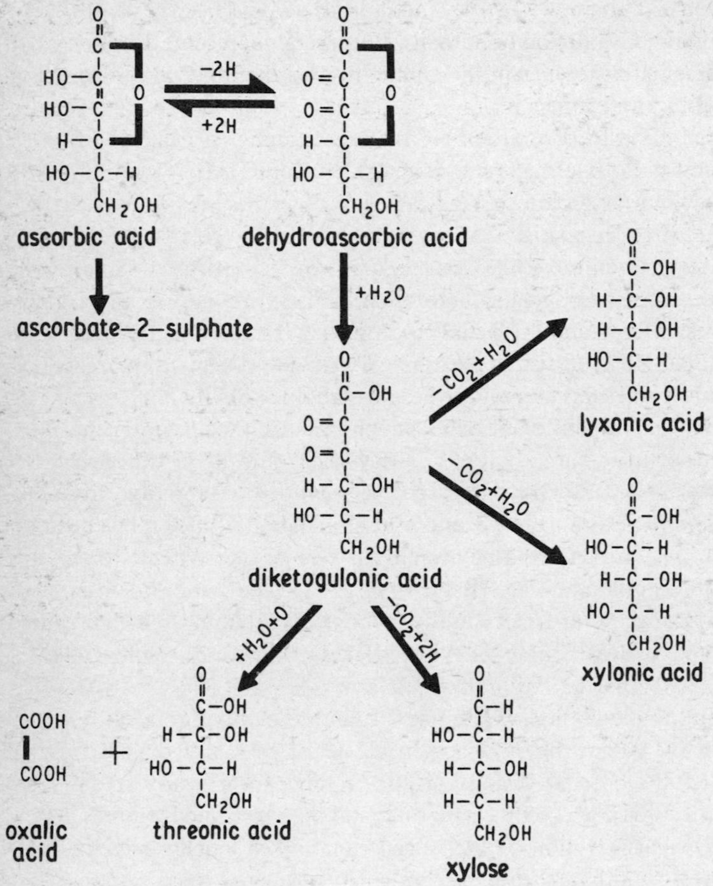

L-ascorbate across the blood–brain barrier, although this is speculative and is based on the observation that free L-ascorbate does not rapidly cross this barrier (Hammerstroem, 1966).

A number of factors are known to affect the way in which vitamin C is catabolised. Thus in scurvy associated with haemosiderosis, the catabolism of the vitamin has been shown to be abnormal. Hanck, Jansen and Schmaeler (1974) provided evidence showing that following ingestion of $(1-^{14}C)$-ascorbic acid by such patients, more than 50 per cent of the radioactivity was excreted in the expired air over a 168-hour period. Usually, only trace amounts of $^{14}CO_2$ are derived from $(1-^{14}C)$-ascorbic acid in the normal adult (Hellman and Burns, 1958; Baker, Saari and Tolbert, 1966) and in experimental scurvy (Baker *et al.*, 1969). In addition labelled oxalate normally represents 50 per cent of urinary radioactivity after $(1-^{14}C)$-ascorbic acid ingestion (Baker, *et al.*, 1962), while in haemosiderotic patients it was found that less than 10 per cent of the total urinary ^{14}C was excreted as oxalate in the first 48 hours. The mechanism by which iron accumulation causes accelerated oxidation of vitamin C to CO_2 awaits clarification.

There has been a number of reports demonstrating that many foreign compounds which cause induction of hepatic microsomal mixed-function oxygenases (Section 3.2.1) also stimulate the urinary excretion of vitamin C in rodents (Conney *et al.*, 1961; Dewhurst and Kitchen, 1973; Tsutsumi, Nakai and Nakamura, 1966). These compounds include nonpolar polycyclic aromatic hydrocarbons, chlorinated compounds and adrenal corticosteroids. It has also been found that these mixed-function oxygenase inducers, such as pheno-barbital which stimulate vitamin C synthesis in the rat, elevate the urinary excretion of D-glucaric acid in man and guinea pigs (Basu and Dickerson, 1974) by inducing the glucaric acid pathway in the liver (Figure 1.1). On the basis of this evidence, it has been suggested that the measurement of urinary vitamin C might be of value in the rat as an indirect index of the activity of hepatic microsomal drug metabo-lising enzymes, and that D-glucaric acid excretion might similarly be used in man and other mammals such as the guinea pig which are unable to synthesise vitamin C.

The validity of these tests to assess drug-metabolising enzyme activity has, however, been questioned. Thus, Aarts (1968) has shown that puromycin and actinomycin D block the stimulation of drug-metabolising enzyme activity but not vitamin C excretion. Furthermore, a lack of correlation between D-glucaric acid excretion and basal rates of drug oxidation has been described (Smith and Rawlins, 1974). Patients on oral contraceptives excrete more D-glucaric acid than the control population, while oral contraceptives do not increase the rate of drug oxidation in man (Mowat, 1968).

It is possible that the oral contraceptives bring about their stimu-latory effect on D-glucaric acid excretion through a mechanism completely independent of the hepatic microsomal enzymes. The chemical basis for how the induction of the mixed-function oxygenases leads to the increase in vitamin C or glucaric acid excretion remains to be established.

1.6 Conclusions

The synthesis of vitamin C and the failure in the process, which results in the compound becoming an essential dietary requirement in man, have been clarified. The details of the breakdown of vitamin C remain to be established. A knowledge of this would clearly be important in our understanding of the way the metabolism of the vitamin seems to be affected by physiological changes, disease processes and drug metabolism (Sections 4.1.2 and 4.2).

2 THE ESTIMATION OF BODY VITAMIN C RESERVES

Since the isolation of vitamin C by Szent-Györgi (1928), numerous attempts have been made to assess body vitamin C reserves, as such measurements have been, and still are, important to our understanding of vitamin C requirements in man. Essentially, researchers are faced with two problems: which method to use for assaying vitamin C and in which tissue or biological fluid to make the measurement.

2.1 Methods Available for the Assay of Vitamin C

Most of the early techniques for measuring vitamin C used the reducing potential of ascorbic acid, the reduced form of the vitamin, to decolourise redox indicators. Many of these techniques are reviewed by Rosenberg (1945). By far the most frequently used indicator has been 2,6-dichlorophenol indophenol originally introduced by Tillmans, Hirsch and Hirsch (1932) and modified by Bessey (1938). The principle of the reaction is illustrated in Figure 2.1. Here ascorbic acid is shown

Figure 2.1: Decolourisation of Dichlorophenol Indophenol by Ascorbic Acid

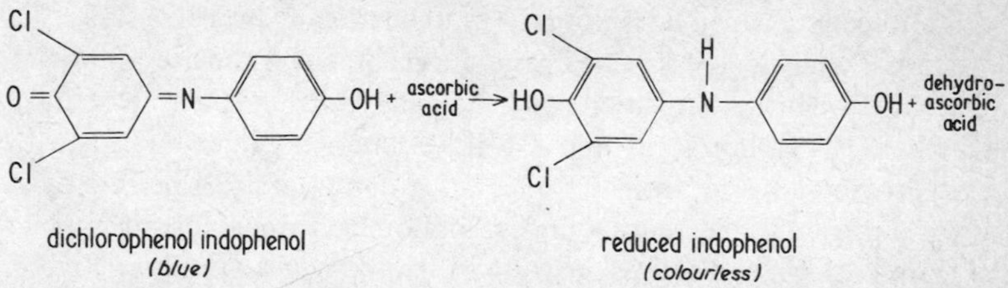

dichlorophenol indophenol
(blue)

reduced indophenol
(colourless)

to reduce the indicator but it is possible for many other reducing agents (e.g. cysteine, sulphides, thiosulphites, ferrous and cuprous ions and reductones produced by cooking) to act in this way (Olliver, 1967a), and hence the technique is potentially unspecific. There is the additional problem that the reagent will only measure ascorbic acid and not the oxidised form of the vitamin, dehydroascorbic acid. It is probable, therefore, that any oxidants such as ferric and cupric ions which oxidise ascorbic acid will give spuriously low readings (Roe, 1954). Furthermore, the dichlorophenol method, whilst rapid and easy, requires a titration which does not have a clear end point. This is reflected in the poor precision of this method especially at low concentrations of vitamin C. Attempts to improve the method have been made by replacing the titration step with a colorimetric measurement (Bessey, 1938), and by increasing the specificity of the assay (Olliver, 1967a). Most procedures use a low pH where relatively few substances reduce indophenol (Roe, 1954). Other modifications have included extraction of vitamin C (Hughes, 1964), the use of formaldehyde (Lugg, 1942), and the combined use of first charcoal to produce dehydroascorbic acid and then homocysteine to reduce, with some degree of specificity, dehydroascorbic acid to ascorbic acid which is then reoxidised by the indophenol dye (Howard and Constable, 1966). Although these techniques increase the specificity of the indophenol method, the extraction procedure increases the risk of loss of vitamin C, whilst the use of other reagents is more time-consuming and still does not ensure absolute specificity for the vitamin.

The reducing potential of ascorbic acid has also been used in reactions with metal ions such as the reduction of ferric to ferrous (Vann, 1965; Zanonni *et al.*, 1974; Day, Williams and Marsh, 1979), and mercuric to mercurous (Kum-Tatt and Leong, 1964) — the reduced metal ion often being coupled with additional reagents — and non-metallic reagents, such as the conversion of 1,2-naphthoquinone by ascorbic acid to its fluorescent dihydro derivative (Hubmann, Monnier and Roth, 1969).

A procedure which does not rely on the reducing properties of vitamin C and which has gained general acceptance is the use of the reagent 2,4-dinitrophenylhydrazine, originally introduced by Roe and Kuether (1943). In this method 2,4-dinitrophenylhydrazine reacts with dehydroascorbic acid, formed from the oxidation of ascorbic acid by oxidising agents added during the estimation, to form an osazone (Figure 2.2) which dissolves in strong sulphuric acid to produce a red colour which is then measured spectrophotometrically. The technique is relatively specific, but estimates not only the biologically active components of vitamin C, ascorbic acid and dehydroascorbic acid, but also the biologically inactive product diketogulonic acid which arises from the oxidation of dehydroascrobic acid (Schaffert and Kingsley, 1955). This is because the hydrazine reagent is capable of forming osazones with any diketone and therefore will act equally well with

Figure 2.2: Reaction of Dehydroascorbic Acid and Sugars with 2,4-dinitrophenylhydrazine

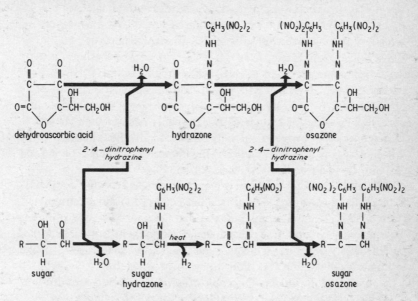

dehydroascorbic acid (produced initially from the ascorbic acid under the reaction conditions used) and diketogulonic acid (Figure 2.2). The hydrazine will also theoretically couple with glucose and other sugars present in biological fluids. However, the oxidation step required following formation of the initial hydrazone with glucose (Figure 2.2) requires heat and under the conditions devised by Roe and Kuether (1943), using a temperature of 37°, the reaction seems specific for compounds of the vitamin C complex (Zloch, Cerven and Ginter, 1971). It should, however, be noted that high molecular weight carbohydrates such as dextran and ficoll (polysucrose), often used to isolate white blood cells before measurement of their ascorbic acid content, can react with the 2,4-dinitrophenylhydrazine reagent to produce substances absorbing at a similar wavelength to the osazone of dehydroascrobic acid. Such interference can usually be avoided if dextran solutions are well drained from the white cell pellets, but in our experience ficoll usually requires washing from the isolated cells with isotonic saline (150 mM/l).

Pelletier (1968) has more recently combined the two most accepted techniques, using the 2,6-dichlorophenol indophenol procedure to measure ascorbic acid and then forming an osazone with the dehydroascorbic acid using 2,4-dinitrophenylhydrazine to measure total vitamin C.

Both the hydrazine and the indophenol techniques, in addition to lacking specificity for biologically active vitamin C, also lack sensitivity. The levels of vitamin C in many human tissues and fluids are so low as to be difficult to measure with precision by either of these methods and even recent techniques still suffer from this problem (Kyaw, 1978; Day, Williams and Marsh, 1979). However, in spite of these problems, both techniques give similar results when used to estimate the plasma vitamin C (Iggo, Owen and Stewart, 1956) and applications of these procedures have probably yielded satisfactory assessments of vitamin C reserves in population studies. This is probably because such large differences occur between the body stores of individuals in many of the different groups studied, and hence high precision has not been needed to show these differences (Sections 4.1 and 4.2).

Details of the hydrazine and indophenol procedures are described by Roe (1954) and Varley, Gowenlock and Bell (1976) and an automated technique has been reported by Garry and Owen (1968). Whilst in the past these procedures have proved adequate, it will be both appropriate and necessary in future to increase the specificity and sensitivity of the estimations of vitamin C in order to be able to measure the individual components of the vitamin C complex (ascorbic acid and dehydro-ascorbic acid) and products of metabolism of the vitamin such as diketogulonic acid. This will be especially necessary when studying vitamin C reserves in hospital populations because acute injury, disease processes and drug metabolism could well affect the relative proportions of the components of the vitamin C complex (Section 4.2). Measurement of these metabolites has already been attempted but it has been questioned whether the techniques used have been adequate (Iggo, Owen and Stewart, 1956). There is also the possibility of drug (e.g. chlorpromazine) interference with current methods and this is important when vitamin C levels are measured in the sick who are receiving drug treatment.

A technique which offers the most potential for increasing the specificity of vitamin C estimations is the use of ascorbate oxidase (Avigliano *et al.*, 1978), an enzyme which in theory could be used in a similar manner to the way glucose oxidase is used to increase the specificity of the measurement of blood glucose concentrations (Morley, Dawson and Marks, 1968). The use of this enzyme is illustrated in Figure 2.3. A number of possible reactions are outlined here, some of which have already been reported. Reaction (a) uses the unspecific reduction of dimethyl-thiazolyl-diphenyl-tetrazolium bromide by ascorbic acid and other reducing agents present in plasma.

Figure 2.3: Potential Use of Ascorbate Oxidase to Measure Ascorbic Acid Concentrations. Reactions (a), (b) and (c) are described in the text.

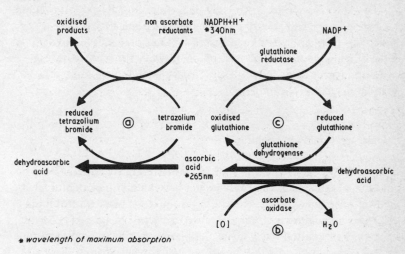

* wavelength of maximum absorption

The reaction is then repeated on another aliquot of the sample after the ascorbic acid has been specifically oxidised by ascorbate oxidase (Reaction (b), Figure 2.3) so only non-ascorbate reductants react with the tetrazolium bromide. Colour produced in the first reaction minus colour produced in the second gives the colour due to the ascorbic acid alone (Boehringer, 1980). Another possible estimation is to convert ascorbic acid to dehydroascorbic acid using ascorbate oxidase (b, Figure 2.3) and then link the re-reduction of the dehydroascorbic acid by glutathione, using the enzyme glutathione dehydrogenase, to the oxidation of reduced nicotinamide adenine dinucleotide phosphate (NADPH) by the oxidised glutathione produced (c, Figure 2.3). The oxidation of the NADPH is followed by a decrease in absorption at 340 nm. However, this is a complex reaction involving several enzymes and in theory there is no reason why the original oxidation of ascorbic acid by ascorbate oxidase (Reaction (b), Figure 2.3) could not be followed by measuring the decrease in optical density at 265 nm, ascorbic acid absorbing strongly at this wavelength ($^E265 = 16.5 \times 10^3 \ 1 \ m^{-1} \ cm^{-1}$ pH7.4, Olliver, 1967c). Whilst this is theoretically possible, in practice other compounds such as amino acids and proteins also absorb at this wavelength and as these are present in biological fluids they ensure very high optical densities at 265 nm. Such problems as the estimation of

small optical density changes at initially very high optical densities
could be handled by sophisticated spectrophotometers, or it may be
necessary to remove some of the absorption due to protein by ultra-
filtration of the sample before assay. It is possible that such procedures
applied in future will greatly increase the speed, specificity and
sensitivity of vitamin C estimations, so that not only will total vitamin
C be estimated but it will be possible to quantify the relative proportions of ascorbic acid, dehydroascorbic acid and diketogulonic acid
within the vitamin C complex.

2.2 Preparation of the Sample

The reduced form of vitamin C (ascorbic acid) is most stable in acid
solution and the majority of researchers have used either trichloroacetic
acid (TCA) or metaphosphoric acid to precipitate unwanted proteins and
achieve acid conditions (Henry, Cannon and Winkleman, 1974). In
our hands plasma and buffy layer preparations stored in 5 per cent
TCA for estimation with 2,4-dinitrophenylhydrazine keep well at
−20° for periods of up to eight weeks. Vitamin C extraction from
tissues should also be made into acid solution to prevent excessive
losses of the vitamin. Roe (1954) recommends the use of TCA for
animal tissues and metaphosphoric acid for plant extracts.

If samples containing vitamin C are not acidified, rapid loss of
ascorbic acid occurs which at neutral pH and 37°C can be as high as
35 per cent in 1 hr (Henry, Cannon and Winkleman, 1974). Because the
rapid oxidation of ascorbic acid results in increases in dehydroascorbic
acid and/or diketogulonic acid, such changes can lead to a spurious
overestimation of these more oxidised compounds. Studies where the
individual components of the vitamin C complex are to be measured
must investigate the effects of collection, preparation and storage of
samples in order to anticipate and prevent artificial changes in the
levels of the vitamin C metabolites under investigation (Roe, 1967).

2.3 Choice of Material for Assessment of Vitamin C Reserves

Most vitamins have been shown to act within the cell quite often
providing essential co-factors for enzyme reactions. Whilst the role of
vitamin C in intermediary metabolism is not fully understood (see
Chapter 3), it seems almost certain that vitamin C will also act

intracellularly probably by modifying or assisting enzyme reactions. Vitamin C will therefore only have biological activity and be effective in an organism when it is presented in the right concentration to the right subcellular site. Whether this is achieved or not will depend upon a number of independent factors. Obviously dietary intake will be important, since an absence of vitamin C in the diet coupled with the inability of the human to synthesise the vitamin will eventually lead to an absence of effective vitamin C at appropriate tissue sites. But between dietary intake and the availability of vitamin C or its metabolites at the site of action within the cell, a number of other factors exert their influence.

These include absorption of the vitamin from the gut, rate of renal excretion, rate of uptake by tissues dependent on vitamin C, rate of metabolism within the tissues and oxidation of vitamin C to its inactive metabolites by infective agents and drugs within the gut, the tissues or the body's fluid compartments. It might well be argued therefore that the best measurement of vitamin C would be a measure of its biological activity at the site of its action. However, Chapter 3 outlines many proposed roles for vitamin C which may have differing degrees of importance for maintenance of health. In addition, these different activities occur in many different tissues. Hence, until the fundamental roles of vitamin C can be determined, measurements of the apparent biological activity of vitamin C in one tissue may not reflect the overall activity of the vitamin in the body. However, some attempts have been made to measure functional vitamin C and these will be discussed later.

Because of these considerations, assessments of vitamin C reserves have largely been confined to a measuremant of dietary intake, concentrations in biological fluids such as plasma, whole blood and urine, and the cellular reserves of the vitamin (Sauberlich, Dowdy and Skala, 1973). More recently, the use of radioactive isotopes of vitamin C has been employed in an attempt to measure the rate of metabolism and the total body pool size of the vitamin. What follows is an assessment of the contributions and limitations of the application of such methods to our understanding of the body's needs for vitamin C.

2.3.1 Dietary Intake

Estimations of dietary intake of a particular component range from the crude dietary recall procedures, where subjects are asked questions of varying detail about their dietary intake, to sophisticated procedures where the actual food is weighed and analysed for the particular component under consideration prior to consumption. Dietary recall procedures are not very dependable (Burke, 1947), but on the other hand are capable of giving an overall idea of dietary intake over a long period of time. In contrast, analysis of food to be ingested is one of the most precise techniques for assessing dietary intake, but this technique is subject to the disadvantage that it can often only be applied over a limited period of time. Provided that there is no suggestion of excessive loss of the vitamin during food preparation, then one of the most satisfactory techniques is that of a weighed dietary intake assessment where subjects weigh their own food and keep a detailed dietary record, usually over a period of seven days (Smithells *et al.*, 1977). Knowing the amount of each food consumed and its composition enables the average daily intake of the principal nutrients to be calculated. Such assessments give a fairly accurate measure of vitamin intake, but are unsuitable for those who, because of limited numeracy and literacy, are unable to carry out a weighed food procedure. Unfortunately it is the diet of these subjects which often deserves the most scrutiny. In addition some individuals may improve their diet during the seven-day assessment in order to hide a poor dietary intake.

Where excessive losses during food preparation are anticipated then some analysis of the vitamin C content of the prepared food should be undertaken. This is particularly important in institutions where food may be maintained at temperatures in excess of 70°C for long periods before serving. Eddy (1968) and Disselduff, Murphy and La (1968) have shown quite conclusively that food in many hospitals contains low quantities of vitamin C due in part to the cooking procedure, a finding which would not have been identified had weighed food assessments been made rather than food analysis. Whilst valuable information, which will be considered later, has been gained by assessment of vitamin C intake, it would seem that future dietary assessments will yield most information when detailed measurements of intake are made in individuals or populations where poor body reserves have been identified and reasons are being sought as to why these poor reserves have arisen.

2.3.2 Plasma Vitamin C

A considerable number of workers have measured plasma or serum vitamin C in an attempt to assess body reserves of the vitamin. This biological fluid is readily available and in theory all vitamin C exchange between the various organs of the body and the transfer of dietary vitamin C to the tissues following its intestinal absorption, must involve the vascular compartment. It is this fact, however, that makes plasma vitamin C reflect recent dietary intake of the vitamin rather than necessarily indicating tissue reserves (Sauberlich, 1975). Following an oral load of the vitamin, plasma levels rise rapidly within one or two hours (Dutra de Oliveira, Pearson and Darby, 1959; Coulehan *et al.*, 1976), probably reaching a peak between 3 and 6 hr (Bordia *et al.*, 1978). Conversely, in times of poor intake the plasma becomes depleted when tissue reserves remain adequate (Crandon and Lund, 1940; Bartley, Krebs and O'Brien, 1953). Plasma vitamin C is also rapidly affected by acute illness (Faulkner and Taylor, 1937; Bartlett, Jones and Ryan, 1940; Crandon *et al.*, 1961; Irwin and Hutchins, 1976; Vallance, Hume and Weyers, 1978). However, rather than being a disadvantage, this may mean that plasma estimations can provide useful information about changes in vitamin C metabolism that can occur during disease.

2.3.3 Tissue Vitamin C

Because the plasma vitamin C concentration is rapidly affected by changes in oral intake, attempts have been made to assess tissue reserves of the vitamin directly. It is fortuitous that leucocytes contain high concentrations of vitamin C, and measurements have been made in these cells in the hope that they reflect overall body vitamin C reserves better than does plasma (Sauberlich, Dowdy and Skala, 1973). There is some evidence that leucocyte vitamin C levels do reflect concentrations in other tissues such as gut and liver, although few such comparisons have been made in the human (Sauberlich, Dowdy and Skala, 1973; Gerson, 1975; Beattie and Sherlock, 1976).

One of the original techniques used for leucocyte separation prior to the estimation of vitamin C in the cells was centrifugation followed by removal of the buffy layer from the surface of the packed red cells (Stephens and Hawley, 1932). More recently, dextran sedimentation of the red cells has been used, a procedure which leaves the platelets and the majority of the leucocytes in suspension (Denson and Bowers, 1961). A modification of the original technique using dextrans of molecular weight greater than 110,000 gives a more satisfactory and rapid sedimentation of the red cells (McCraw and Sim, 1969). Centrifugation of the supernatant left after dextran sedimentation yields a buffy layer, which is a mixture of white cells contaminated with platelets (Gibson, Moore and Goldberg, 1966; Attwood *et al.*, 1974). Vitamin C is almost invariably expressed as the concentration per number of leucocytes and rarely are contaminating platelet levels taken into account. Platelets in a typical buffy layer contain high concentrations of vitamin C equivalent to those found in the leucocytes (Gibson, Moore and Goldberg, 1966). Failure to allow for platelet contamination leads to error in the estimation when there are differences in the ratio of leucocytes to platelets between buffy layers prepared on different occasions. It is probable that failure to take account of the contribution of platelets in the buffy layer could be in part responsible for the inverse relationships between leucocyte numbers in the buffy layer and leucocyte vitamin C concentration (Vallance, 1979; Evans, Currie and Campbell, 1980). A theoretical example of how such a relationship could arise can be seen when increasing numbers of white cells, each containing the same amount of vitamin C, are obtained from different preparations, but with each preparation containing the same number of platelets. In order to achieve an expression of the vitamin C concentration in terms of a given number of leucocytes (usually 10^8), the fractions with the greater number of leucocytes would have their total vitamin C (leucocyte + platelet) multiplied by a smaller factor than those where the number of leucocytes were less. Hence, correction for the increasing number of leucocytes maintains a constant and correct value for the leucocyte concentration but the quantity of platelet and therefore total vitamin C is artificially decreased.

However, this artificial effect is only part of the explanation for the negative relationship between leucocyte number and their vitamin C concentration. There is also a negative correlation between leucocyte vitamin C and leucocyte numbers in whole blood, as opposed to buffy layer (Maclennan and Hamilton, 1976), which although in part being artificially induced by the platelet contribution mentioned above (Evans, Currie and Campbell, 1980), is probably also influenced by physiological change. Vitamin C is decreased in leucocytes in acute disease or trauma when there is often an associated rise in blood leucocyte number (Barton, Laing and Barisoni, 1972; Hume *et al.*, 1972; Hume and Weyers, 1973; Irvin, Chattopadhyay and Smythe, 1978). It is suggested that this reflects either a sharing of available vitamin C throughout the increased number of leucocytes (Vallance, 1979) or a migration of vitamin C rich leucocytes into areas of damage to be replaced by vitamin C poor polymorphic leucocytes (Maclennan and Hamilton, 1976; Vallance and Hume, 1979). This 'injury' response makes the leucocyte vitamin C less able to reflect overall tissue reserves of the vitamin and a correction for leucocyte number by expressing leucocyte vitamin C as the quantity in the leucocytes/ml of blood (Griffiths, 1968; Schorah *et al.*, 1978), rather than the quantity/ unit number of leucocytes, may be a more valid way of assessing the tissue reserves of individuals whose blood white cell numbers are changing. The final problem lies in the heterogeneity of the white cell population where neutrophils and lymphocytes may also contain different quantities of vitamin C (Stankova *et al.*, 1977).

In order to overcome these difficulties it has been suggested that correction factors could be applied (Gibson, Moore and Goldberg, 1966), but it is now possible to separate the individual-cell fractions (Pertoft, Back and Lindahl-Kiessling, 1968) and it would seem appropriate in future that, wherever possible, assessment of tissue vitamin C reserves is made not on a buffy layer but on either platelet, lymphocyte or neutrophil vitamin C or on all three fractions. For the reasons mentioned above, such estimations will be particularly important when vitamin C levels are measured in subjects who are ill, where the leucocyte and platelet numbers may vary greatly from subject to subject or are changing rapidly within an individual. Even then care should be taken to standardise separation procedures which will minimise the exchange of vitamin C between the cells and plasma.

Studies attempting to separate the buffy layer components have suggested that the platelets and leucocytes contribute approximately equally to the buffy layer vitamin C (Attwood *et al.*, 1974). In healthy subjects the platelets have an average concentration ranging from $1-7$ μg/10^9 cells (Barkhan and Howard, 1958; Lloyd *et al.*, 1972; Attwood *et al.*, 1974; Sarji, Kleinfelder and Brewington, 1979) and the leucocytes $11-22$ μg/10^8 cells (Barkhan and Howard, 1958). Within the leucocyte population the concentration of vitamin C in the lymphocytes is approximately double that found in the polymorphic neutrophils (Thomas and Holt, 1978). There are approximately 4×10^9 platelets per 1×10^8 leucocytes in the buffy layer preparation (Attwood *et al.*, 1974) which would give a calculated range for the buffy layer vitamin C of $15-50$ μg/10^8 leucocytes. This is close to the reported reference ranges for buffy layer vitamin C (Chapter 4) which suggests that the separate analysis of the buffy layer components are giving approximately the correct values. Few studies have measured platelet-free leucocyte vitamin C and researchers that have used buffy layer measurements always express them as leucocyte vitamin C. Consequently, in this book leucocyte vitamin C will be used as a synonym for buffy layer and where platelet-reduced or free leucocyte preparations are assessed these will be clearly indicated.

Leucocyte (buffy layer) preparations are obviously technically more complex than plasma and may be impractical in large studies. There is, however, a relationship between plasma and leucocyte vitamin C (Figures 4.1 and 4.2). For individuals the relationship is not linear and shows a wide scatter (Lowry *et al.*, 1946; Griffiths *et al.*, 1967). This is shown clearly in Figure 4.1, where it is apparent that in a number of subjects plasma concentrations fall to very low levels whilst leucocyte vitamin C remains adequate. Conversely, leucocytes appear to reach saturation whilst plasma vitamin C continues to rise. It is likely, therefore, that a plasma estimation would be an unsatisfactory measure of vitamin C tissue reserves for individuals, especially if there has been a recent change in dietary intake which might occur on admission to hospital. However, when the relationship between the mean leucocyte and the mean plasma vitamin C of populations is examined (Figure 4.1) it is clear that there is a close, almost linear relationship. This might be expected as the variations in individuals are largely eliminated. For population studies it seems, with hindsight, that plasma vitamin C has reflected leucocyte and therefore tissue vitamin C and thus may be used in large studies where resources do not allow for vitamin C estimations to be made on the buffy layer or on the individual cell types, and where sudden changes in dietary intake or metabolism of vitamin C are not anticipated.

When individuals are to be assessed for vitamin C depletion then leucocyte (buffy layer) estimations, provided that there are no gross increases in leucocyte or platelet numbers, should be able to identify those at risk of clinical scurvy who will have very low leucocyte levels (less than $10\mu g/10^8$ cells, Chapter 4). Identification of individuals who have suboptimal reserves (Chapter 4), but are not frankly vitamin C deficient, is more difficult in the absence of adequate cell separation procedures and repeat analysis of both plasma and leucocyte vitamin C may be necessary to establish a correct baseline for these patients.

2.3.4 Assessment of Biological Turnover and Body Pools of Vitamin C

The most frequently applied technique used to assess these parameters has been the study of the rate of excretion of the reduced form of vitamin C (ascorbic acid) in the urine of subjects who have been given a large oral dose of the vitamin. A number of studies have indicated that the ability of the renal tubule to reabsorb vitamin C filtered through the glomerulus is exceeded when plasma vitamin C rises to 0.75–1.0 mg/100 ml, and this leads to rapid loss of the vitamin in the urine (Figure 2.4) (Friedman, Sherry and Ralli, 1940; Kallner,

Figure 2.4: Loss of Vitamin C in the Urine as Plasma Concentrations Rise Above the Threshold for Tubular Reabsorption. The shaded area indicates the approximate 95 per cent range.

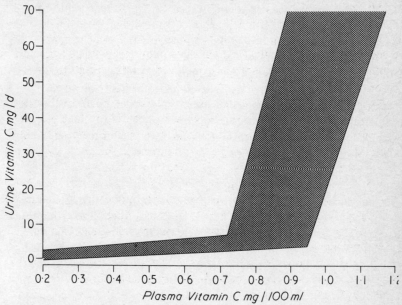

Hartmann and Hornig, 1979). If vitamin C reserves in the body are low, then an oral dose will not increase plasma vitamin C sufficiently to allow loss of ascorbic acid in the urine. On the other hand, as vitamin C reserves increase then a large oral dose of the vitamin will lead to the threshold of renal reabsorption being approached and eventually exceeded, resulting in increasing losses of vitamin C in the urine. Hence, the lower the body saturation or the greater the rate of vitamin C metabolism, the larger will be the oral intake required to bring about a loss of a significant quantity of vitamin C in the urine. Measurement of the intake required to bring about significant urine loss gives an assessment of tissue status. This technique is often referred to as a vitamin C saturation test and details of the procedure are described by Varley, Gowenlock and Bell (1976). It is probable that such a test will give unreliable information in subjects who have reduced renal function, such as the elderly and the sick (O'Sullivan *et al.*, 1968).

More recently, attempts to measure reserves and the rate of metabolism of vitamin C have relied upon the use of radioactive isotopes of ascorbic acid. The rate of disappearance of the isotope from the plasma and its excretion in the urine along with the measurement of total vitamin C in these two compartments, allows an assessment of rate of metabolism and the body pool size of vitamin C and also speculation about the various compartments into which vitamin C can enter. Such studies have been undertaken during tissue depletion and repletion of vitamin C (Baker *et al.*, 1971) and during steady-state conditions where vitamin C intake and reserves are held constant (Kallner, Hartmann and Hornig, 1977). Although such techniques often require the hospitalisation of the subjects under study for several days if not weeks, and the calculations made inevitably involve a number of theoretical assumptions, such studies will be invaluable in the future in assessing changes in vitamin C metabolism which appear to occur during disease processes (Section 4.2) and during drug therapy (Rivers and Devine, 1975).

2.3.5 Attempts to Measure the Biological Activity of Vitamin C

Some of the earliest attempts to measure vitamin C were assessments of the effectiveness of samples on the treatment of artificially induced scurvy in experimental animals (Olliver, 1967a). Such techniques are rarely used today as they are time-consuming and expensive, requiring vitamin depletion in large numbers of animals in order to overcome the biological variation inherent in such assays.

Vitamin C has long been implicated in the synthesis of collagen where it is believed to be involved in the hydroxylation of proline and lysine residues after their incorporation into procollagen polypeptide chains (Section 3.1.1). In vitamin C deficiency the reduction in the rate of this hydroxylation is believed to lead to the accumulation of the unhydroxylated precursor-collagen polypeptide chains which cannot be effectively utilised and are subsequently broken down and their amino acids either re-utilised or excreted in the urine. This produces two effects: there is a decrease in the excretion of hydroxylated proline and lysine whilst the levels of the unhydroxylated forms increase. Urine measurements of the ratio of the unhydroxylated to hydroxylated forms have been used in a number of studies to assess vitamin C reserves (Windsor and Williams, 1970; Bates, 1977). There is however recent evidence that such measurements are an insensitive assessment of vitamin C status (Bates *et al.*, 1979). This may be because the unhydroxylated procollagen molecules are unable to be glycosylated, are therefore not released from the cell and thus inhibit further synthesis of procollagen molecules (Barnes and Kodicek, 1972).

Another proposed biological role for vitamin C is its involvement in the synthesis of the free fatty acid carrier carnitine (Hulse, Ellis and

Henderson, 1978). Hughes and associates have measured the levels of muscle carnitine in guinea pigs during vitamin C depletion and have found low levels. They further suggest that such measurements may be of practical importance in the human for assessing the biological activity of the vitamin (Hughes, Hurley and Jones, 1980). Less invasive plasma carnitine assays are available (Mitchell, 1978) and may be more appropriate in the human.

Tyrosine excretion following an oral dose of the amino acid has been used by Crandon and colleagues (1958) to assess the vitamin C status of surgical patients. The test does not measure a physiological role of the vitamin (Section 3.2.7), but following large oral intakes tyrosine excretion seems to reflect differences in vitamin C reserves, although the test is technically difficult requiring the collection of a three-day urine sample.

Vitamin C has been implicated in a number of other biological roles in the human (Chapter 3) and it is feasible that a reduction in the potential of any of these systems could be used as a measure of decreasing vitamin C reserves.

2.3.6 Conclusions

In the past, most studies have relied on the measurement of plasma and more recently leucocyte vitamin C to assess body reserves of the vitamin. Evidence would suggest that the leucocyte measurement, at any rate in population studies, adds little additional information to our knowledge gained from the measurement of plasma levels. In individuals this may not be true since fluctuations in dietary vitamin C rapidly affect plasma concentrations. However, it is not necessarily true that the leucocyte measurement in the individual would have contributed much to our understanding of an individual's vitamin reserves because of the known errors in the leucocyte (buffy layer) assessment when the concentration of vitamin C in platelets that contaminate the preparation is not taken into account. As will be discussed later, it is probable that in future we will wish to measure vitamin C reserves in populations where either acute or chronic diseases are affecting the metabolism of the patient. Under these conditions it will be necessary to assess vitamin C reserves using a tissue measurement and here it would seem appropriate to attempt to measure the levels in the individual buffy layer components separately (i.e. platelets, neutrophils and lymphocytes). An estimation of a rate of turnover of vitamin C, probably by measuring the distribution and excretion of isotopically labelled vitamin C, will also be important in

Figure 2.5: Suggested Scheme of Assays Required for a Better Assessment of Body Vitamin C Reserves

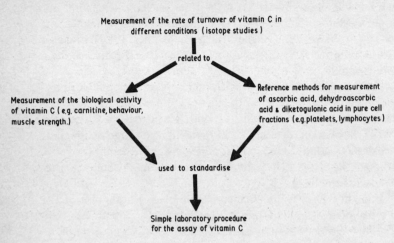

these studies. Where this is impractical or unethical, the excretion of vitamin C in the urine during an oral load would give some idea of increased or decreased metabolism of vitamin C.

It is essential that all the studies should be undertaken using an accurate method for assessing the vitamin C level in the biological material chosen. This may require the separate estimation of the biologically active components of vitamin C, ascorbic acid and dehydroascorbic acid, and in addition the estimation of the first inactive metabolite of vitamin C, diketogulonic acid.

Such accurate assessments of vitamin C reserves and turnover would be of limited value without the means to relate the findings to biochemical, physiological and clinical changes which occur during vitamin C depletion. Hence, it will be necessary to have some measurement of the biological activity of vitamin C, such as the measurement of muscle or plasma carnitine levels.

Most of these techniques would be reference procedures. It would be difficult and inappropriate to apply them to large population surveys or day-to-day diagnostic services. It will therefore be necessary to compare the results of the reference method with the values found by a simpler technique, such as a plasma vitamin C estimation, so that the simpler technique can be applied on a wider scale, such as in a service laboratory. Here the relatively rapid and simple procedure of Day, Williams and Marsh (1979) may be of use if it proves robust and specific in routine use. An outline of these suggestions is presented in Figure 2.5.

3 THE ROLE OF VITAMIN C

The only role of vitamin C which has been categorically established is the ability of the vitamin to prevent and cure clinical scurvy. It is beyond the scope of this book to discuss in detail the clinical aspects of scurvy, but an outline would be appropriate. General features include swollen joints, muscular aches and bone pain, oedema, weakness, fatigue, anaemia and hyperkeratosis, especially around the hair follicles. In severe cases, there may be failure of wounds to heal and even a breakdown of scar tissue with the reopening of old wounds (Anson, 1748). There are also behavioural changes which are characterised by apathy, depression and emotional disturbances and a number of characteristics which are probably related to a weakening of the walls of blood vessels, for example swollen and bleeding gums, ocular haemorrhages, bruising, petechial haemorrhages and dilations, or more correctly varicosities, of small blood vessels which are seen under the tongue. Not all these symptoms are seen in every patient. For further details of clinical scurvy, the reader is referred to the following: Lind (1753); Cutforth (1958); Goldberg (1963); Walker (1968); Hodges *et al.* (1971); Wilson (1975); Eddy and Taylor (1977).

The full clinical condition is rarely seen today except in the elderly, where in industrial areas the incidence can be as high as 1 per cent (Exton-Smith, 1980). Whilst clinical scurvy is uncommon, there is considerable evidence that low body vitamin C reserves can occur in a relatively large proportion of the population without the clinical symptoms being manifest, although it has been suggested that some of the signs and symptoms associated with the disease may be present. Some workers believe that this condition, often called chronic sub-clinical vitamin C deficiency or hypovitaminosis C, has metabolic and clinical features different from acute clinical scurvy (Turley, West and Horton, 1976; Ginter, 1979a) and leads directly to impaired health and to increased susceptibility to other disease. These suggestions, many of which are controversial, will be considered further in Chapters 4 and 5, but clarification of the situation would be simplified if we had a better understanding of the metabolic function of vitamin C. It is the purpose of this chapter to consider critically the evidence for the proposed metabolic roles of the vitamin.

Elucidation of the role of vitamin C can be approached in two ways, either by a study of the enzymes and the biochemical reactions in which the vitamin is believed to be involved, or by an investigation of the clinical signs and physiological disturbances which appear as the tissues become depleted of the vitamin. The former leads more directly to the actual role, but such studies are often undertaken with isolated cells or purified enzymes and there is difficulty in establishing the significance of these findings in the whole animal. The latter, in contrast, reflects more closely the physiological situation, but the evidence is often more difficult to interpret. Whilst many roles have been suggested, those where evidence from one of the above approaches can explain findings from the other are most likely to indicate a true physiological function for the vitamin. It is these we will examine in most detail, but others will be considered because, as indicated above, there is controversy about the sub-clinical signs of C deficiency, and hence some suggested biochemical functions of vitamin C may apparently lack clinical expression because the clinical signs are not yet recognised as part of the symptoms of C deficiency.

We will try and avoid roles which have been attributed to the vitamin following studies in animals subjected to extreme depletion of C, where starvation and approach of death causes many metabolic disturbances which are probably due to deficiency of many essential nutrients in addition to the primary depletion of C (Ginter, 1979a).

3.1 Vitamin C as a Reducing Agent

The redox potential for the reduction of dehydroascorbic acid to ascorbic acid is +0.080 V (White *et al.*, 1978) and this would place the vitamin in the position indicated in the redox chart shown in Table 3.1. Here electrons will flow down the redox charge gradient from top to bottom so that each compound is chemically capable of reducing any substance below it. Hence, in equimolar concentrations, vitamin C can be reduced by reduced NAD or glutathione, but will itself reduce cupric ions, ferric ions, the metal ions bound to many of the body's cytochromes and oxygen. The reactions are purely chemical and need not have any significance in biological systems, but some of the enzymes involved in these reactions have been identified, although not all have been found in human tissues, and these are illustrated in Figure 3.1. The presence of enzymes suggests a physiological role for these reactions; however, their significance is as yet unknown, although it would seem that reactions (a) and (b) probably help to return vitamin

Table 3.1: Reduction Potentials for Vitamin C and Substances Capable of Reacting with the Vitamin in Biological Systems

Reaction	Redox Potential for Reaction (volts)
Nicotinamide adenine dinucleotide $\rightarrow$ reduced nucleotide	−0.32
Oxidised glutathione $\rightarrow$ reduced glutathione	−0.23
Dehydroascorbic acid $\rightarrow$ ascorbic acid	+0.08
$Cu^{++} \rightarrow Cu^{+}$	+0.15
Cytochrome $a_3 \rightarrow$ reduced cytochrome	+0.39
$Fe^{+++} \rightarrow Fe^{++}$	+0.77
Oxygen $\rightarrow H_2O$	+1.23

C to the reduced form after its oxidation by reactions (c), (d) and (e) or other enzymes not yet identified (Figure 3.1). There is now considerable evidence that some of these unidentified enzymes capable of oxidising ascorbic acid may be oxygenases some of which appear to require ascorbic acid as a reducing agent.

3.1.1 Vitamin C and Oxygenases (Hydroxylases)

Oxygenases are classified according to the type of reaction they catalyse (Hayaishi, Nozaki and Abbott, 1975). There are dioxygenases where both molecules of oxygen are incorporated into one substrate or, as in the case of vitamin C dependent enzymes, two separate substrates. The action of this last group, the intermolecular dioxygenases, can be described by the following formula where Sub_I and Sub_{II} are the two substrates to be oxygenated

$$O_2 + Sub_I + Sub_{II} \xrightarrow[\substack{\text{reducing} \\ \text{agent} \\ Fe^{++}}]{} Sub_I{-}O + Sub_{II}{-}O \qquad (Eq. 3.1)$$

It seems to be a requirement in all the intermolecular dioxygenases so far identified for one of the substrates to be 2-oxoglutarate, and so the equation can be rewritten

$$O_2 + \text{2-oxoglutarate} + Sub_{II} \xrightarrow[\substack{\text{reducing} \\ \text{agent} \\ Fe^{++}}]{} \text{succinate} + CO_2 + Sub_{II}{-}O \qquad (Eq. 3.2)$$

Figure 3.1: Enzyme Systems (a–e) Oxidising and Reducing Compounds in the Ascorbic Acid Complex. The broken line represents possible oxidation of ascorbate by several oxygenases described in Section 3.1.1

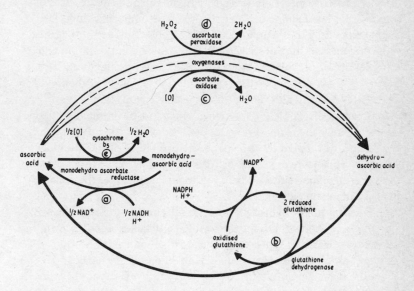

One atom of oxygen appears in the new carboxyl group of succinate, the other is in the other substrate, usually in a hydroxyl group. The requirement for ferrous ions is specific but a number of substances can fulfil the role of the reducing agent (Hayaishi, Nozaki and Abbott, 1975), although for several enzymes ascorbic acid seems to be the best *in vitro* hydrogen donor. The function of the reducing agent may be either to maintain the iron in the ferrous state or, along with ferrous ion, to induce the production of a highly active form of oxygen, such as superoxide, which can then attack the substrates directly.

The other type of oxygenase is the mono-oxygenase where only one atom of oxygen is incorporated into the substrate, the other being reduced to water with the help of a hydrogen donor which can be either the substrate itself or an external reducing agent. In the latter case, the oxygenases are called mixed-function oxygenases and for at least one of these mono-oxygenases the hydrogen donor is ascorbic acid, although there is some evidence that vitamin C may be involved with other mixed-function oxygenases.

Proline and Lysine 2-oxoglutarate Dioxygenases. These two enzymes,

often called prolyl and lysyl hydroxylases, are responsible for hydroxylating the amino acids proline and lysine once they have been
incorporated into polypeptide chains. Apart from elastin, which
contains a few residues, only collagen contains significant amounts of
these hydroxylated amino acids and so the most important function
of these enzymes is in the hydroxylation of these residues in the three
polypeptide chains of procollagen prior to triple helix formation and
before release of procollagen from the cell (Barnes and Kodicek, 1972;
Barnes, 1975). A number of the hydroxylysine residues are then
glycosylated and this aids release of the procollagen from the cell
(Barnes and Kodicek, 1972), following which loss of terminal polypeptide units allows the formation of tropocollagen and then subsequent
cross-linking of these residues leads to the formation of the insoluble
collagen fibres (White *et al.*, 1975). It is at this final stage that
hydroxyproline molecules are believed to add stability to the collagen
molecule (Rao and Adams, 1979).

The mechanism of hydroxylation is similar to that outlined in
Equation 3.2. There is considerable evidence that the reducing agent in
both hydroxylation of lysine and proline is the reduced form of
vitamin C, ascorbic acid. Consequently, in vitamin C deficiency, it is
believed that the amount of effective collagen fibre present in
connective tissue is reduced. This is due to a reduced rate of hydroxylation which in part decreases the number of hydroxylysine residues
and lowers the rate of synthesis of procollagen (Barnes and Kodicek,
1972) and also makes the collagen fibres less stable through a reduction
in their hydroxyproline content.

However, although ascorbic acid would appear to be the most
effective reductant, there is evidence that other hydrogen donors will
also react (Barnes and Kodicek, 1972; Hayaishi, Nozaki and Abbott,
1975) and these include vitamin C analogues such as isoascorbate
(Miller, Elsas and Priest, 1979), although this latter compound has
little biological vitamin C activity in the whole animal (Hornig, 1977).
It has also been suggested that depletion of the vitamin only leads to a
partial reduction in collagen synthesis (Barnes and Kodicek, 1972) and
hence the slow development of the lesions of scurvy which require
between 60 to 100 days of vitamin C deficiency to develop (Bartley,
Krebs and O'Brien, 1953; Hodges *et al.*, 1971). Indeed, it has been
reported that the cell responsible for collagen synthesis, the fibroblast,
can in culture hydroxylate proline in the absence of vitamin C,
although addition of the vitamin enhances the hydroxylation (Priest
and Bublitz, 1967). Finally, an inborn error of metabolism (Ehlers-

Danlos syndrome, type VI) leads to a deficiency of lysyl hydroxylase which results in a replacement of hydroxylysine by lysine in the procollagen fibres. This change however leads to connective tissue disorders which are not characteristic of scurvy (McKusick, 1974), although there is some evidence that vitamin C can modify the condition (Elsas, Hollins and Pinnell, 1974).

In spite of this contrary evidence, recent work has shown that in highly purified preparations of prolyl hydroxylase, ascorbic acid is the essential reductant and other reducing agents will not substitute (Tuderman, Myllyla and Kivirikko, 1977). It appears to be oxidised to dehydroascorbate during the reaction, but not in a one-to-one relationship with the number of hydroxyproline residues formed. Evidence would suggest that the ascorbic acid acts as a specific agent for maintaining the activity of the enzyme by reducing the ferric ion, which tends to be formed in the reaction, back to the active ferrous state required by the enzyme (Myllyla, Kuutti-Savolainen and Kivirikko, 1978).

Such studies are of course far removed from the physiological situation found in the cell, but it has long been recognised that some of the lesions of scurvy can be explained by a change in connective tissue metabolism (Gould, 1963). The gum and bone changes and failure of wounds to heal could arise from a reduction in the amount of collagen fibre formed. The tendency of blood vessels to haemorrhage could also be explained by a weakness in the connective tissue structure of their walls (Booth and Todd, 1972; Eddy and Taylor, 1977). Differences in the signs of Ehlers-Danlos syndrome from those of scurvy may be explained by evidence which suggests that vitamin C may not only be important in hydroxylation, the enzyme lesion in the syndrome, but also in the formation of collagen fibres outside the cell (Candlish and Tristram, 1963; Gould, 1963), synthesis of the components of the ground substance of connective tissue, the mucopolysaccharides (Gould, 1963; Nambisan and Kurup, 1975; Ginter, 1979a), and maturation of fibroblasts (Ross and Benditt, 1964), the cells responsible for collagen and mucopolysaccharide production.

In biochemical terms, there are decreases in the excretion of hydroxyproline and hydroxylysine in the urine of individuals suffering from vitamin C depletion with increases in proline and lysine, suggesting a physiological role for the vitamin in amino acid hydroxylation, although this is not considered a sensitive marker of vitamin C depletion (Section 2.3.5).

Overall, evidence suggests that vitamin C probably acts as an important and specific reducing agent for the proline and lysine dioxygenases (hydroxylases). Vitamin C depletion produces a defective connective tissue, although this may be slow to develop due to the very small quantities of vitamin C which are able to maintain hydroxylation or to the ability of other reducing agents to substitute, albeit less effectively, for vitamin C in this particular dioxygenase reaction.

Dioxygenase Reactions in Carnitine Biosynthesis. There is evidence that vitamin C is essential for two steps in the synthesis of muscle carnitine (Hulse, Ellis and Henderson, 1978). Both these reactions are hydroxylation steps and again involve intermolecular 2-oxoglutarate dioxygenase enzymes and follow the reaction mechanisms outlined in Equation 3.2. As with the amino acid hydroxylases, there is evidence that other reducing agents e.g. tetrahydrofolate can replace vitamin C as co-factor for the butyro-betaine-2-oxoglutarate dioxygenase, the final step in carnitine synthesis. However, clinical evidence would suggest an essential role for vitamin C in these reactions. Carnitine is required for transfer of fatty acids into the cells' mitochondria where they can be used for energy production. Low carnitine concentrations, which have been found in the muscles of vitamin C-depleted guinea pigs, should lead to poor energy production and muscle weakness which Hughes, Hurley and Jones (1980) believe accounts for the symptoms of fatigue and lassitude seen in scurvy in man (Lind, 1753; Crandon, Lund and Dill, 1940; Bartley, Krebs and O'Brien, 1953; Kinsman and Hood, 1971). There is also evidence that tissue saturation with high-dose vitamin C leads to some increase in athletic performance in the human, although it must be emphasised that such improvements are marginal (Howald and Segessar, 1975) and smaller supplements are said to have no effect in overall physical efficiency in labourers (Fox *et al.*, 1940).

Dopamine β-mono-oxygenase. One of the copper containing mono-oxygenases, this enzyme is responsible for the hydroxylation of dopamine to noradrenalin. The mechanism is different from the dioxygenase reaction in that ascorbic acid would appear to be a direct hydrogen donor rather than protecting the enzyme from inactivation. The hydrogen from ascorbic acid is used to reduce to water the atom of oxygen not incorporated into the dopamine (Ullrich and Duppel, 1975). The copper atom in the enzyme acts as an intermediate, accepting electrons from ascorbate as it is reduced to the cuprous ion and subsequently transferring these electrons to oxygen as it is

reoxidised back to the cupric ion (Figure 3.2). Evidence would suggest
that ascorbate cannot be effectively replaced by other reducing agents
(Kaufman and Friedman, 1965) and its importance in this step in the
synthesis of noradrenalin and adrenalin may explain the need for
specific and active transport mechanisms which concentrate vitamin C
from the plasma through the spinal fluid into the brain cells and account
for the high levels found in the adrenal gland (Section 1.3). This process
guarantees that the brain cells remain adequately supplied with vitamin
C even when plasma levels fall (Spector, 1977).

**Figure 3.2: Possible Mechanism for the Dopamine Mono-oxygenase
(DMO) Reaction. Recent work suggests monodehydro-ascorbic acid as
the initial product of vitamin C oxidation.**

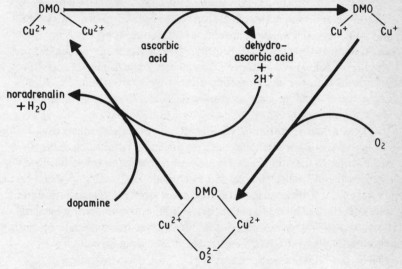

Source: Adapted from Ullrich and Duppel (1975).

If vitamin C is important in the synthesis of brain amines, and there
is evidence to suggest that C status effects amine synthesis *in vivo* in
animals (Deana *et al.*, 1975), one would expect neurological disorders
to develop when there were inappropriate amounts of the vitamin in
nerve tissue. Animal studies have indicated that vitamin C injected into
the brain is able to affect dopamine function (Tolbert *et al.*, 1979)
possibly by increasing its metabolism to noradrenalin. The vitamin also
has an inhibitory effect similar to the neurotoxin 6-hydroxydopamine
which destroys the dopamine system of the rat brain leading to a

decrease in its dopamine content (Waddington and Crow, 1979). Alternatively, when biologically active amines are injected into the brain they appear to cause an increase in the level of vitamin C in those areas where they are injected (Subramanian, 1977).

These studies have led to the suggestion that vitamin C therapy may be of advantage in conditions such as schizophrenia, chorea and diskinesia, which are conditions of dopamine excess (Tolbert *et al.*, 1979). Certainly, depression is a feature of scurvy (Cutforth, 1958; Walker, 1968) and there is evidence that patients with chronic schizophrenia (Akerfeldt, 1957; Vanderkamp, 1966) and other bahavioural disorders (Kinsman and Hood, 1971; Irwin and Hutchins, 1976) have low vitamin C reserves in their plasma and leucocytes. Indeed, in a placebo trial, Milner (1963) showed that supplementation with vitamin C brought about an improvement in patients with depression and schizophrenia. He further suggested that these patients had an increased demand for vitamin C, a finding supported by Hoffer and Osmond (1967) who believe that the vitamin is utilised in the removal of toxic metabolites such as adrenochrome. However, Pitt and Pollitt (1971) were unable to find either low reserves or an increased demand for the vitamin in schizophrenics carefully matched with the control groups.

There would seem to be little dispute about the role of vitamin C in the synthesis of noradrenalin, but it is unclear whether deficiency of the vitamin in the brain cells can be severe enough to cause the common diseases which lead to changes in behaviour, such as schizophrenia and depression. To distinguish cause and effect from mere association in these conditions, it will be necessary to undertake research which will overcome the many problems which arise when studying patients with psychiatric disease. These include: the heterogeneous nature of psychiatric disease and the necessity for precise classification of patients under study and the selection of appropriate controls and double-blind procedures; the fact that chronic disease can lead independently to both behavioural changes and poor nutrition and that poor dietary intake will often occur in untreated psychiatric disease; the difficulty of establishing appropriate and valid psychometric tests which will detect change during treatment; and finally the problem that a psychiatric patient is often prescribed several drug preparations which can not only have their rate of excretion changed by vitamin C but also affect both the rate of metabolism (Section 3.2.1) and the assay of the vitamin (unpublished observations).

3.1.2 Other Reducing Functions of Vitamin C

Reduction of Folic Acid. Anaemia is common in scurvy (Goldberg, 1963; Vilter, 1967). Whilst there are many possible reasons for this, for example blood loss through haemorrhage, lack of iron uptake and increased destruction of the red cell (Goldberg, 1963), it is clear that a number of patients who are suffering from scurvy have a megaloblastic anaemia which is due to an effective deficiency of folic acid (Stokes *et al.*, 1975). This leads to an inability to synthesise sufficient nucleic acid and red cell production is decreased accompanied by the release of abnormal red cells, the megaloblasts, into the circulation (Vilter *et al.*, 1963). Some of these patients respond to vitamin C, a few require folate (Cox, 1968). Stokes and co-workers (1975) present evidence in one patient that the megaloblastic anaemia associated with scurvy is caused by an inability to maintain folic acid as the reduced tetrahydro-folate, the active form of the vitamin, this metabolite being rapidly metabolised to the more oxidised folic acid which is then excreted in the urine. Vitamin C appeared to prevent this oxidation and led to a rapid correction of the anaemia. It has also been noted that decreased vitamin C leads to an increase in urinary folic acid excretion which can be corrected by vitamin C therapy (Booth and Todd, 1972). The possible role of ascorbic acid in maintaining the stability of tetrahydro-folate (Figure 3.3) was originally suggested by Nichol and Welch (1950) and re-emphasised by Vilter and co-workers (1963), but more recently Banerjee and Nandy (1970) have found that the guinea pig deficient in

Figure 3.3: Outline of Folic Acid Metabolism. The reduced active metabolites of folate, indicated with asterisks, are protected by vitamin C, the monoglutamate being rapidly excreted.

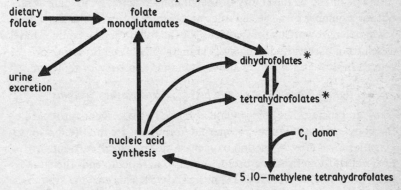

vitamin C is still able to carry out conversion to tetrahydrofolate quite adequately. In the human, it has been noted that there is an association between plasma and leucocyte vitamin C levels and folic acid concentrations (Exton-Smith, 1980; Bates *et al.*, 1980). This could mean that one vitamin affects the metabolic availability of the other or alternatively that a dietary source poor in one vitamin is also poor in the other and therefore deficiencies of folate might arise in association with, but metabolically independent of, vitamin C depletions. Indeed, Bates *et al.* note that vitamin C supplementation had no effect on folate levels in patients with low concentrations of both vitamins.

Available evidence would suggest that at best vitamin C depletion is only important in folate metabolism in isolated situations. Such situations could arise in advanced disease where multiple deficiencies are common and folate levels are low in association with a reduced supply of many nutrients such as those vitamins (nicotinic acid, riboflavin, vitamin B_{12} and vitamin C) whose metabolites could be involved in aiding folate reduction or maintaining tetrahydrofolate levels. Such a situation could arise in pregnancy where multiple marginal deficiency of folate, vitamin C and vitamin B_{12} may collectively reduce cell growth in the fetus and contribute to the causation of the neural tube malformations, spina bifida and anencephaly (Smithells, Sheppard and Schorah, 1976; Schorah, Smithells and Scott, 1980; Smithells *et al.*, 1980).

3.2 Other Roles of Vitamin C

It would seem reasonable to expect that all functions of vitamin C would be linked to the ability of the vitamin to act as a reducing agent, but for a number of suggested roles no obvious redox mechanisms have as yet been shown. Such suggestions for the function of vitamin C have arisen from observation of changes in metabolites, cell function, or general health resulting from either vitamin C depletion or repletion.

3.2.1 Vitamin C and Cytochrome P450 Hydroxylating Systems

Many drugs and other lipid-soluble potentially toxic agents produced by the body, such as bilirubin and steroid hormones, are modified prior to excretion by a mixed-function oxygenase system which is found predominantly in liver microsomes but also in reticulo-endothelial tissues throughout the body (Lehninger, 1975). This enzyme system requires a number of components which include enzymes for hydroxylating and demethylating substrates, flavoproteins, a cyto-chrome protein (P450), oxygen and the provision of reducing agents, usually in the form of reduced NADP or NAD. A diagrammatic representation of the reactions involved is shown in Figure 3.4.

Figure 3.4: Liver Cytochrome P450-dependent Mixed-function Oxygenase. Levels of P450 and the oxygenase are increased by vitamin C.

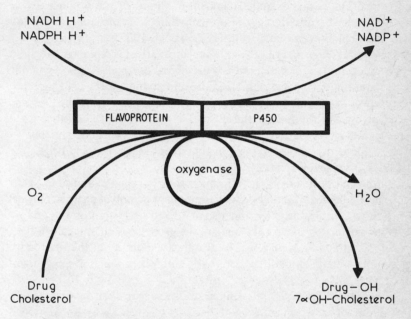

There is considerable evidence linking changes in the activity of this mixed-function oxygenase with changes in vitamin C status. Theoretically, this role of the vitamin should be included in the oxygenase section above, but there is no evidence that vitamin C is either involved directly in the hydroxylation process, as it is in the dopamine mono-oxygenase, or in maintaining iron in the reduced form, as in dioxygenase reactions. Animal studies have suggested that depletion of vitamin C is associated with a decrease in the activity of many of the enzymes involved in these reactions and also a decrease in the actual quantity and stability of the microsomal electron transport system, cytochrome P450 (Degkwitz *et al.*, 1975; Fielding and Hughes, 1975; Zannoni, 1977; Zannoni and Sato, 1975, 1976; Rikans, Smith and Zannoni, 1978). Not only does vitamin C deficiency apparently lead to a decrease in these components, but there is also an association between the level of vitamin C reserves and the rate of metabolism of drugs both in animals (Conney *et al.*, 1961; Street and Chadwick, 1975) and in the human (Rosenthal, 1971; Beattie and Sherlock, 1976). In patients with liver disease, the slowest rates of drug metabolism were found in those with the lowest vitamin C concentrations (Beattie and Sherlock, 1976), although liver disease itself leads to a decrease in vitamin reserves (Bonjour, 1979) and can obviously also lead to a decrease in drug metabolism by that organ independent of vitamin C status. Such findings have led to the suggestion that vitamin C supplements may be required in diseases that affect the liver (BMJ, 1977).

Not only does vitamin C status appear to affect the rate of drug metabolism, but increased rates of drug breakdown also change vitamin C status, increasing its synthesis in the rat (Conney *et al.*, 1961) and its turnover in the guinea pig (Street and Chadwick, 1975). In the human, an example of this may be the changes in vitamin C metabolism and decreases in plasma and leucocyte concentrations which are seen in those patients who are taking oral contraceptives (Briggs and Briggs, 1975; Irwin and Hutchins, 1976).

The exact role of vitamin C in microsomal drug metabolism has yet to be elucidated. Is it an essential component or only a pharmacological stimulant, activating in a manner similar to the way barbiturates and some organopesticides will stimulate the process? A pharmacological role for vitamin C is suggested by the apparent ability of the vitamin to stimulate metabolism of cholesterol by this mixed-function oxygenase.

Cholesterol Hydroxylation. Animal studies suggest that the first step in cholesterol excretion and its conversion to bile acids is hydroxylation at the 7α position on the steroid nucleus (Figure 3.5) by the liver microsomal cytochrome P450-dependent mixed-function oxygenase (Wada *et al.*, 1968, 1969). Whilst vitamin C does not appear to enhance the activity of this mixed-function oxygenase directly (Kritchevsky, Tepper and Story, 1973; Bjorkhem and Kallner, 1976), marginal vitamin C depletion in the guinea pig leads to a reduction in the activity of this rate-limiting step in cholesterol metabolism (Ginter, 1973, 1978; Hornig and Weiser, 1976), probably by a decrease in the components of the microsomal mixed-function oxygenase system as described above (Degkwitz *et al.*, 1975; Zannoni and Sato, 1975; Bjorkhem and Kallner, 1976; Ginter, 1979a). This reduction in the cholesterol-hydroxylating capacity of the animal's liver (Bjorkhem and Kallner, 1976) leads to an increase in tissue (including arterial) and/or

Figure 3.5: Detail of the Initial Step in Cholesterol Oxidation

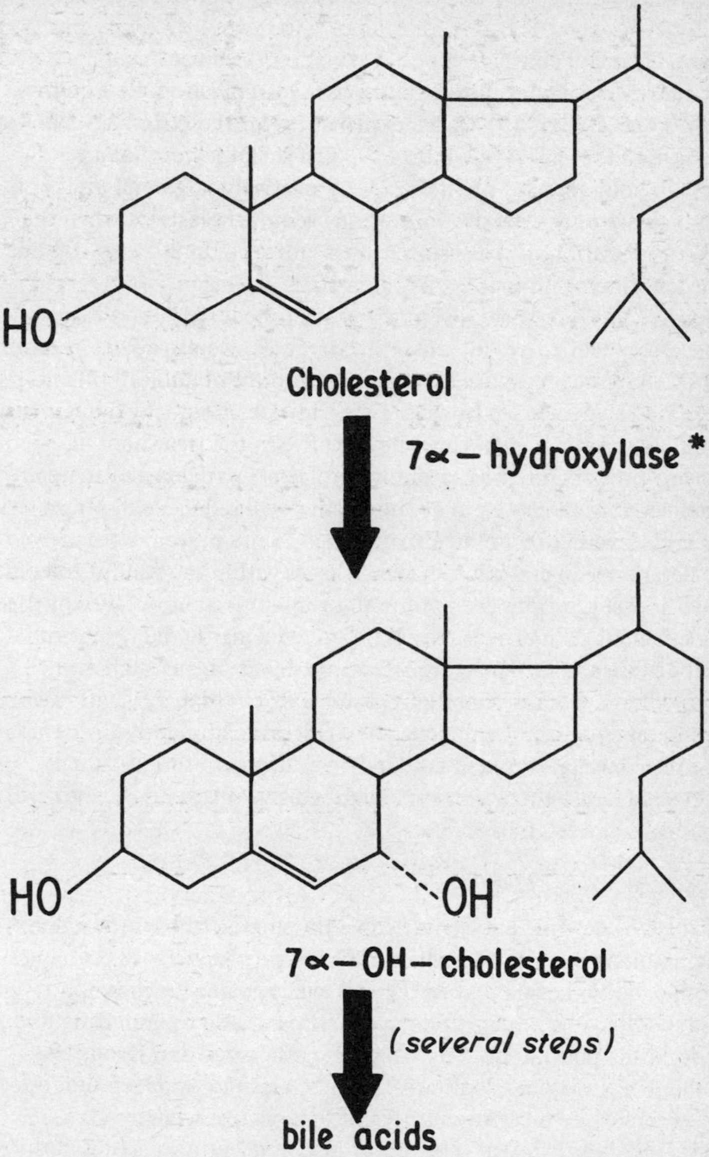
HO
Cholesterol
7α – hydroxylase *
HO
OH
7α–OH–cholesterol
(several steps)
bile acids

* *levels are decreased in vitamin C depletion*

serum cholesterol (Ginter, 1973, 1975; Ginter, Babala and Cerven, 1969; Ginter *et al.*, 1967; Hornig and Weiser, 1976; Nambisan and Kurup, 1975).

There are many conflicting publications on the association between vitamin C reserves and serum cholesterol in man (Turley, West and Horton, 1976; Ginter, 1978). An explanation for these findings has been suggested recently by Ginter (1979b). He indicates that an increase in body reserves of vitamin C by relatively large oral intakes of the vitamin are only effective in lowering serum cholesterol when the initial concentration of the serum lipid is greater than 200 mg/100 ml. In a review article, Ginter (1979a) also draws attention to the mixed aetiology of hypercholesterolaemia and the probability that vitamin C will be largely ineffective in controlling hypercholesterolaemia in those patients who have a primary defect in the control of cholesterol synthesis (Brown and Goldstein, 1974). However, there is evidence that appropriate vitamin C intake can be effective in the treatment of a reasonable proportion of hypercholesterolaemic patients and there are also publications indicating that the vitamin will reduce high serum triglyceride levels, affect clotting mechanisms and prevent connective tissue deterioration and micro-haemorrhages within the wall of arterial tissue. These suggestions are potentially very important because of the possible benefit such effects may have on reducing the incidence of arterial disease and its damaging effects on major organs such as the heart and brain. Because the findings are controversial and, with the exception of cholesterol and collagen changes, lack underlying biochemical mechanisms and convincing evidence to support them, and often advocate the use of very high intakes of vitamin C, they will be considered in detail in Section 5.2.

3.2.2 Cyclic Nucleotides

Lewin (1976) devoted a relatively large proportion of his monograph to championing the idea that vitamin C was able to increase both cyclic adenosine monophosphate (cAMP) and cyclic guanosine monophosphate (cGMP) by increasing their synthesis, and also by inhibiting the 3,5-nucleotide phosphodiesterase enzyme (Malamud and Kroll, 1980) which destroys these nucleotides. There is certainly evidence that cGMP levels are increased in tissue cultures of monocytes, neutrophils and lymphocytes in the presence of rather high concentrations of ascorbic acid or the calcium and sodium salts of ascorbate (Sandler, Gallin and Vaughan, 1975; Anderson, 1979; Atkinson *et al.*, 1979). Such changes in cyclic nucleotides, if they occur under physiological conditions, could have a multitude of effects as it is known that these nucleotides are synthesised when hormones bind to their specific cell receptors and act as mediators of hormone action (Cramer and Schultz, 1977).

One such effect could be in the asthmatic patient, where it has been suggested that decreased vitamin C may be in part responsible for the condition (Olusi *et al.*, 1979) by decreasing cAMP levels and hence leading to increased histamine release (Lewin, 1976). There is recent evidence that increased intake of vitamin C can relieve both experimental and clinical asthma (Zuskin, Lewis and Bouhuys, 1973; Anah, Jarike and Baig, 1980). It has also been suggested that the effects of vitamin C on dopamine (Section 3.1.1) in nerve tissue may be mediated through changes in cyclic nucleotides (Tolbert *et al.*, 1979). However, rather than increasing cAMP, vitamin C has been shown to inhibit the dopamine-stimulated increase in the cyclic nucleotide in animal brain cell homogenates, and this action of the vitamin mimics that of the antipsychotic drug haloperidol (Thomas and Zemp, 1977).

Clearly as yet there is little firm evidence that vitamin C is directly implicated in increasing cyclic nucleotide concentrations. Indeed the effect could be indirect, as vitamin C is required in the synthesis of noradrenalin and adrenalin (Section 3.1.1), hormones which themselves could affect the cAMP levels of their target organs (Skolnick and Daly, 1977).

3.2.3 Metabolism and Absorption of Iron

There is evidence in both animals and humans that vitamin C can affect the distribution of iron and its storage protein ferritin between the tissues and the plasma. In vitamin C deficiency, increasing quantities of iron are deposited in the tissues and serum levels of iron and ferritin bear little relationship to tissue iron reserves. The correlation can be restored by tissue C repletion (Wapnick, Bothwell and Seftel, 1970; Roeser *et al.*, 1980). Vitamin C is also said to increase the intestinal uptake and peripheral metabolism of iron (Prasad, 1975). Alternatively, pure iron deficiency anaemia in children leads to higher vitamin C reserves, whilst subsequent iron therapy, although not affecting plasma vitamin C, reduces cellular levels (Bingol *et al.*, 1975) and iron overload accelerates oxidation of C (Lynch *et al.*, 1967). Because of these associations, vitamin C has been used to increase the absorption of iron from iron-fortified milk (Stekel, 1980). However, 500 mg a day of vitamin C in the diet did not improve the response of anaemic women to iron, folic acid or vitamin B_{12} in a recent study in India (Mathen *et al.*, 1979) and it seems unlikely that the anaemia seen in scurvy in many individuals is due mainly to iron deficiency (Goldberg, 1963). It would seem therefore that whilst vitamin C may be able to influence iron uptake from the gut, and affect its tissue distribution, the role of vitamin C in iron metabolism and particularly in promoting haemoglobin synthesis in iron-deficiency anaemia, remains unresolved.

3.2.4 Vitamin C and Sulphation

In the human, vitamin C is in part metabolised to ascorbic acid-2-sulphate (Section 1.5). Although some of this sulphated ascorbate is excreted in the urine, a proportion may be used to sulphate other compounds such as cholesterol (Verlangieri and Mumma, 1973) and components of connective tissue, the mucopolysaccharides (Gould, 1963; Nambisan and Kurup, 1975). Cholesterol sulphation may aid its excretion, although it is unknown to what extent this occurs under physiological conditions, and sulphation of mucopolysaccharides is important in the formation of connective tissue, although the need for ascorbic acid in this reaction is not firmly established.

3.2.5 Prostaglandins and Vitamin C

There is very little evidence for a role of vitamin C in prostaglandin synthesis in man, but some very recent reports have suggested that high levels of C can increase the synthesis of prostaglandins in isolated platelets and cells in tissue culture (Horrobin, Oka and Manku, 1979; Polgar and Taylor, 1980). Horrobin and colleagues (1979) have further hypothesised that this role in prostaglandin metabolism could explain many of the functions of vitamin C. This awaits experimental confirmation.

3.2.6 Immunological Effects of Vitamin C

The study of the body's immunity to infective agents is a subject in its own right (Roitt, 1977), but essentially the immune response to foreign material occurs through the following mechanisms. The first is the production of specific protein antibodies to the infective agent (antigen), such antibodies being either cell bound on sensitised lymphocytes (cell-mediated immunity) or free antibody released into the blood by β-lymphocytes, which mature in the bone marrow (the humoral-mediated immunity). Binding of these antibodies to the antigen along with proteins of the complement complex, also produced by lymphocytes, not only neutralises bacterial toxins, but also aids the action of less specific immune mechanisms, the ingestion and killing of bacteria by phagocytic cells such as the neutrophils. It is these cells, the neutrophils and the lymphocytes, which are involved in the immune response, which together form a large proportion of the white cell population of the blood.

Here then is the most obvious link between immunity and vitamin C; the cells that are responsible for the immune response contain very high concentrations of vitamin C of the order of 40 to 60 times the concentration found in the plasma (Section 1.3). These high concentrations within the leucocytes are rapidly depleted by acute disease, infection and trauma (Section 4.2.1). In addition, a number of chronic diseases and conditions which lead to a depression of immunity such as cancer, diabetes, ageing, corticosteroid therapy and pregnancy are also associated with low levels of plasma and leucocyte vitamin C (Chapter 4). Together, these associations have led researchers to look for a role for vitamin C in the immune response.

With the exception of work by Vallance (1977) and Prinz *et al.* (1977) who indicate that there is some association between leucocyte and plasma ascorbic acid levels and immunoglobin components (the humoral antibodies), there is little evidence that vitamin C stimulates the humoral side of the immune response. So research has concentrated on lymphocyte-mediated immunity and the phagocytic activity of the neutrophil.

Much of the earlier work has been with animal cells and has shown an involvement of vitamin C in the migration of phagocytes and changes in the metabolism of the lymphocyte. References to much of this work are included in the review by Thomas and Holt (1978). Recently, a number of studies on the human have been reported. In a number of papers (Goetzl *et al.*, 1974; Sandler, Gallin and Vaughan, 1975; Anderson, 1979; Anderson and Theron, 1979a,b) it has been shown that vitamin C in fairly high concentrations is able to stimulate neutrophil motility, increase cGMP levels and promote the glycolytic activity of the cell *in vitro*, changes which are believed to reflect the ability of the neutrophil to attack bacteria. This has been confirmed and extended to show that vitamin C appears to have this effect on both random migration of the neutrophil and also on true chemotaxis, that is movement of the neutrophil in the presence of and along a gradient of the stimulating agent (Dallegri, Lanzi and Patrone, 1980). Lymphocytes are also stimulated by ascorbic acid *in vivo* but possibly not *in vitro* (Anderson, Oosthuizen and Gatner, 1979; Ramirez *et al.*, 1980), their transformation to blast cells, the precursor of the effector cell in both cell-mediated and humoral immunity, being accelerated by the vitamin. In addition, the inhibition of this transformation by influenza viruses is corrected by large doses of vitamin C (Manzella and Roberts, 1979).

Partial *in vivo* studies, where vitamin C is given to individuals and the effect of this is studied later in the isolated white cells, have confirmed these *in vitro* findings. Under these conditions, vitamin C appears to stimulate both transformation of the lymphocyte (Yonemato, Chretien and Fehniger, 1976; Anderson *et al.*, 1980) and neutrophil motility (Anderson *et al.*, 1980; Rebora, Dallegri and Patrone, 1980). In support and confirmation of these findings some patients with a defective immune response who suffer repeated infections, thought to be primarily due to poor neutrophil function, have responded well to large doses of vitamin C, their improved clinical condition paralleling improvement in the behaviour of their isolated neutrophils (Anderson and Dittrich, 1979; Rebora, Dallegri and Patrone, 1980). Although there has been a number of studies which have suggested little or no effect of vitamin C on these white cell parameters (Shilotri and Bhat, 1977; Gallin *et al.*, 1979), the positive evidence would now seem significantly to outweigh the negative findings.

The actual metabolic role of vitamin C in these cell changes is unknown, although it appears to stimulate glucose metabolism in human cells (Shilotri and Bhat, 1977; Anderson, 1979). Recent work has suggested that the neutrophil, when in contact with bacteria, generates superoxide on the surface of the cell using reduced NADP to reduce the oxygen as indicated below (Babior, 1977).

$$NADPH + H^+ + 2O_2 \longrightarrow NADP^+ + 2O_2^- + 2H^+ \qquad \text{(Eq. 3.3)}$$

The wall then invaginates to form an intracellular vacuole containing the bacteria and surrounded by membrane capable of creating super-oxide which can then attack and kill the bacteria aided by lysosomal enzymes which also enter the vacuole (Johnston and Lehmeyer, 1977; Roos *et al.*, 1977).

Ascorbate would appear to have no direct role in this process as the free energy for the reaction is not favourable, the redox potential for the reduction of oxygen to superoxide being -0.33 V. (As mentioned earlier that for ascorbate reduction is $+0.080$ V.) Superoxide is however highly toxic, so much so that within the neutrophil there is an enzyme, superoxide dismutase, carrying the unfortunate abbreviation SOD, which prevents damage to the cell by encouraging destruction of the superoxide that escapes from the vacuole containing the ingested bacteria:

$$2O_2^- + 2H^+ \longrightarrow H_2O_2 + O_2 \qquad\qquad \text{(Eq. 3.4)}$$

This reduction of superoxide to peroxide however has a redox of +0.9 V and hence can in theory be performed by ascorbic acid (Nishikimi, 1975):

$$2O_2^- + \text{ascorbic acid} + 2H^+ \longrightarrow 2H_2O_2 + \text{dehydroascorbate}$$
$$\text{(Eq. 3.5)}$$

There is evidence that at concentrations found within the neutrophil ascorbate may play a significant part in the removal of superoxide, complementing the activity of SOD (Nishikimi, 1975). Indeed, as SOD is intracellular, superoxide escaping from the neutrophil could damage surrounding tissue and cause inflammatory disease (Johnston and Lehmeyer, 1977). Vitamin C, unlike the enzyme, is not limited to the cell and could serve as a protective agent to surrounding tissues.

Alternative proposals for the role of vitamin C in the immune response have suggested that it can contribute to bacterial killing by aiding production of the toxic hydroxyl free radical (Bjorksten, 1979). Stimulation of interferon production by human lymphocyte and fibroblast cultures has also been noted to occur in the presence of vitamin C (Siegel, 1975; Stone, 1980).

Whilst we remain uncertain of the actual role of vitamin C in the white cells, as Thomas and Holt (1978) conclude in their review, there is now considerable evidence that vitamin C is involved in the immune response and therefore in protection against infection. This certainly seems to be the case in a small number of individuals who appear to have a suppressed immune response and suffer from repeated infections (Anderson and Dittrich, 1979; Anderson and Theron, 1979b). Most interest has, however, concentrated on the effectiveness or otherwise of vitamin C in combating respiratory and other viral infections (e.g. the common cold), and as these treatments often require high intakes of the vitamin they will be considered further in Section 5.1.

3.2.7 Roles Now Considered of Little Significance

Two effects which at one time were thought to be important in human metabolism now seem unlikely roles for the vitamin. One of the earliest biochemical effects noted was a fall in adrenal vitamin C in the rat when the gland was stimulated by ACTH (adrenocorticotrophic hormone) (Seyers *et al.*, 1946). Although some of the metabolic steps in steroid hormone synthesis are hydroxylation steps which in theory could involve vitamin C (Section 3.1.1), no function for vitamin C in steroid hormone metabolism in man has been found. The adrenal responds normally to ACTH and steroid excretion is often normal in scorbutic human subjects (Woodruff, 1964).

Metabolism of tyrosine was also believed to involve vitamin C, since abnormally high plasma tyrosine levels and urine concentrations of its metabolite *p*-hydroxyphenyl pyruvic acid could be decreased by giving C to scorbutic infants and to both adults and premature infants receiving large intakes of tyrosine (Woodruff, 1964). It is now clear that ascorbic acid does not function as a necessary factor in tyrosine metabolism, but protects the enzyme *p*-hydroxyphenyl pyruvate oxidase from inhibition by its substrate under the artificial conditions of high tyrosine intake (La Du and Zannoni, 1961). In this situation vitamin C can be replaced by other reducing agents. The vitamin can however be used to treat tyrosinaemia in the premature infant (Levine, 1947).

3.3 Conclusions

A summary of the present position for suggested roles of vitamin C based on the available evidence is presented in Table 3.2. The involvement of vitamin C in the dioxygenase reactions resulting in hydroxylation of the amino acids lysine and proline has been suspected for many years, but more recently it has been found to be important in other hydroxylation processes that occur in the synthesis of carnitine and noradrenalin. Debate continues as to whether the requirement for vitamin C is absolute in these reactions, but both biochemical and clinical evidence would suggest that either this is the case or that in the absence of the vitamin the reaction mechanisms are far less efficient. It would seem however, that relatively small quantities of the vitamin are required for these processes to operate and that in the case of the synthesis of amines in the brain and adrenal glands, specific transport mechanisms guarantee that the cellular concentrations of the vitamin are maintained in the presence of relatively low serum levels. This is illustrated by the relatively long periods of vitamin depletion that are required in the human (30–100 days) before lesions which could be related to a disturbance of the underlying biochemical mechanisms develop: connective tissue damage—decreased amino acid hydroxylation; lethargy and muscle weakness — reduced carnitine levels; behavioural disturbances — inappropriate brain amine concentrations. Of course there are few studies on the human, and it may be that

Table 3.2: Suggested Roles of Vitamin C Grouped by Strength of Current Evidence

---

Considerable evidence that vitamin C directly involved:
    Vitamin C essential:
        Proline and lysine hydroxylation
        Carnitine synthesis
        Dopamine hydroxylation

    Vitamin C aids or affects, but not essential (may be required in high concentrations):
        Drug and cholesterol breakdown
        Sulphation
        Lymphocyte and neutrophil function
        Folate reduction
        Iron distribution

Little evidence that vitamin C directly involved:
    Interferon production
    Prostaglandin synthesis
    Cyclic nucleotide metabolism
    Glucose metabolism

---

careful clinical assessment of behaviour and detailed histological studies of connective tissue might reveal earlier changes than have yet been observed. Certainly, experimental depletion has, for ethical reasons, been undertaken in healthy subjects and there is evidence that disease leads to a more rapid depletion of the body's vitamin C reserves.

Whatever the tissue level of vitamin C required for hydroxylation, evidence for other roles of the vitamin have been reported. These, such as the maintenance of microsomal drug and cholesterol metabolism and its suggested role in cellular immunity, may well not be essential functions in the way that an enzyme has an absolute requirement for a co-factor. The vitamin could provide a bonus, aiding other substances, such as other reducing agents, in their role in these mechanisms. Although acting as an ancillary agent, vitamin C could be important in maintaining health through such roles, in a similar manner to the way in which oil and petrol additives can reduce wear and improve the performance of a car. Thus the human body may be more susceptible to and less able to recover from disease and in the long term suffer degenerative change more readily in the absence of an adequate supply of the vitamin.

An adequate supply of the vitamin is difficult to define, but if it has a preventive role then reserves must be readily available to meet any increased need which infection, imbalance of diet, use of alcohol, smoking, drugs or social stress could induce (Ginter, 1979a). Hence, supporters of such a role for vitamin C have suggested that very high intakes may be required for the vitamin to be effective in this way. These intakes are many times greater than the recommended, and are above those which will keep the tissues of a healthy individual saturated. Such suggestions are speculative, but there are reports indicating benefit from high intake in conditions such as arterial disease, viral infection and cancer, conditions where decreased cholesterol breakdown or poor immune response could be implicated. These hypotheses can be coupled with the increasing concern that, for many in our society, not only are tissues far from saturated with the vitamin, but that some, especially those in hospital, have low reserves which for a few approach those seen in clinical scurvy (Schorah, 1979).

In the next chapter, we shall therefore examine critically how detrimental to our health poor tissue reserves may be and what intakes are required to maintain appropriate vitamin C concentrations, whilst in Chapter 5 we will consider how effective large intakes of vitamin C are in combating disease.

4 VITAMIN C RESERVES AND REQUIREMENTS IN HEALTH AND DISEASE

It is the purpose of this chapter to examine the range of vitamin C reserves found in man and to consider their significance in relation to physical and mental health. It is, however, important to emphasise that it will not be possible to be certain about our predictions, since considerably more research must be undertaken before definitive answers can be proposed. Nevertheless, we believe that there is sufficient evidence to make some provisional suggestions. It is not anticipated that the same intake will be required to achieve adequate body stores in all subjects. This is because change in intake, which can be influenced by factors such as season and social class, is not the only way in which vitamin C reserves can be affected, although it probably makes the most important single contribution. A number of parameters such as state of health, drug therapy and sex can influence vitamin C reserves by changing the metabolism of the vitamin. Some of these components may also affect vitamin C intake as well as metabolism. It will therefore be appropriate, initially, to examine the way these factors can influence both intake and/or metabolism of vitamin C.

There are as yet no completely satisfactory ways for assessing the vitamin C reserves of individuals without recourse to complex metabolic studies using isotopes (Chapter 2). However, assessments of the way vitamin C reserves are influenced can be made by comparing the mean values for vitamin C calculated from measurements made by relatively simple techniques in subjects grouped by the factors under consideration e.g. sex, age or state of health. The techniques which have been used most frequently are plasma and leucocyte (buffy layer) vitamin C. Not all studies have used both techniques, however, and it will therefore be necessary to examine the relationship between these two measurements. Figure 4.1 shows such a relationship. Here the mean values for different populations of adults we have studied are shown along with the 95 per cent range of the individual results. It is quite clear that the scatter when individual values are plotted is enormous. For example it is possible for two individuals to have the same plasma value of 0.30 but leucocyte levels which range from 5 to 40 $\mu g/10^8$ cells. In contrast, mean values for plasma and leucocyte vitamin C show a close relationship. The wide scatter of individual results serves to emphasise

Figure 4.1: Relationship between Plasma and Leucocyte Vitamin C. Mean values for several populations are indicated by the symbols; the lines show the 95 per cent range for individual results.

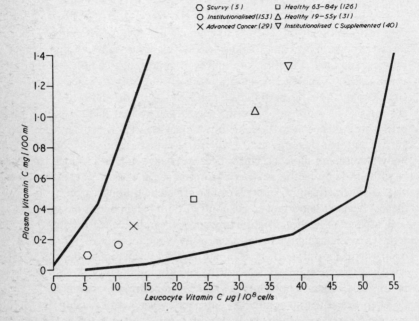

POPULATION GROUP AND NUMBER IN GROUP

○ Scurvy (5)   □ Healthy 63–84y (126)
○ Institutionalised(153) △ Healthy 19–55y (31)
✕ Advanced Cancer (29) ▽ Institutionalised C Supplemented (40)

that the assessment of C concentrations in an individual is difficult and indicates that estimations by several different techniques may be required in order to establish the approximate body reserve of a patient. Figure 4.2 shows the 95 per cent range of mean values found in over thirty publications taken randomly from the literature over the last forty years. The data are limited to subjects who were living in industrialised and developed nations and who were not suffering from acute disease (values for institutionalised populations where the majority of patients were suffering from psychiatric disease, dementia or paralysis are included). The spread of results is now wider than the mean values from our own studies (Figure 4.1), but it is clear that the relationship between mean plasma and leucocyte vitamin C, as assessed by many different laboratories, is remarkably close. This re-emphasises the point made in Chapter 2 that for population studies, the mean plasma values probably reflect vitamin reserves as well as the more complex leucocyte estimations.

Figure 4.2: Ninety-five per cent Range of the Mean Values for Plasma and Leucocyte Vitamin C Reported in Over Thirty Publications During the Last Forty Years

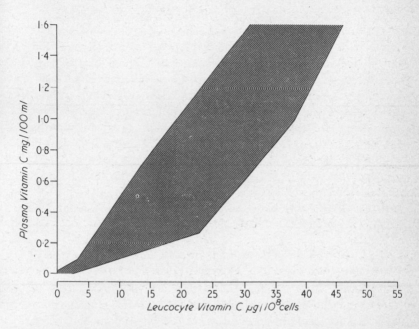

As there is evidence that leucocyte measurements reflect tissue and therefore whole body vitamin C reserves (Chapter 2) and as mean plasma levels are closely related to those in the leucocyte, both plasma and leucocyte concentrations reported in this chapter will be assumed to reflect whole body vitamin C status. Where there are exceptions to this rule, such as conditions which might cause a rapid shift of vitamin C between the vascular compartment and the tissues, these will be indicated.

Within the leucocyte and plasma relationship considerable differences occur between different population groups, some having high reserves whilst others have almost no measurable vitamin C (Figure 4.1). What factors influence these variables and produce such wide differences in leucocyte and plasma vitamin C concentrations between population groups, and what reserves are needed to maintain health? We shall consider the first question initially and the second in Section 4.3.

4.1 Factors which Affect the Level of Plasma and Leucocyte Vitamin C in Health

Factors affecting plasma and leucocyte vitamin C can essentially be divided into two categories, those that influence metabolism and those that influence intake of the vitamin. In developed nations vitamin C intake is largely determined in the healthy by food preference and its preparation, rather than on the availability of the food. Quite clearly intakes will vary considerably from individual to individual but such variation, if random throughout the population, would not explain the differences in the population groups seen in Figure 4.1 which, in the unsupplemented, range from the younger healthy group down through the elderly and those with chronic disease to the institutionalised and those with clinical scurvy. These groups must therefore differ in either intake or metabolism of vitamin C or both. Whilst there is some overlap between the influence of these two effects, some differences in C reserves can be largely explained on the basis of changes in one or the other.

4.1.1 Differences in Plasma and Leucocyte C Determined by Different Intakes

Most soft fruit and vegetables are a good source of vitamin C (Olliver, 1967b) and a balanced diet should provide reasonable intakes of the vitamin. There are however two limiting influences. Although there are many foods available with a reasonable vitamin C content, some people choose not to eat a balanced diet and in addition vitamin C is arguably more susceptible than any other essential nutrient to destruction and loss during the storage and preparation of the food. Storage of vegetables can lead to losses of up to 80 per cent (McCance and Widdowson, 1960; Olliver, 1967b; Millross *et al.*, 1973) probably through oxidation by a variety of enzymes present in the plant cells. Oxidation losses also occur in preparation and cooking when slicing and crushing can encourage oxidation, especially if there is delay before the ascorbate oxidases are inactivated by heat (Olliver, 1967b; Millross *et al.*, 1973), and most cooking procedures lose vitamin C through some leaching of the vitamin from the food especially during boiling (Olliver, 1967b). Finally, one of the major causes of vitamin C loss in institutions occurs after cooking when the food is kept hot for long periods.

In some cases overall losses are so extreme that less than 10 per cent of the vitamin C in the fresh food reaches the consumer (Streightoff *et al.*, 1949; Eddy, 1968; Glew, Hill and Millross, 1971).

Such are the losses in institutionalised food, that new cook-freeze methods of preparation have been proposed in an attempt to retain the nutrient value of the food during preparation (Millross *et al.*, 1973). Currently, however, such is the potential for loss of the vitamin from food that it is not surprising that it is possible to identify sections of the community where vitamin C tissue reserves differ largely because of differences in intake.

Social Class. The Registrar General's social class groupings (Office of Population Censuses and Surveys, 1970) are at best a very crude assessment of family wealth and dietary habit in the UK. However, populations classified by these groupings do show differences in vitamin C reserves (Schorah *et al.*, 1978; Moore, Rohatgi and Low, 1979) and socio-economic groups show similar trends in other countries (Chope and Dray, 1951; Morgan, Gillum and Williams, 1955). Exton-Smith (1980) has also shown regional differences in plasma vitamin C concentrations, although there was little difference in the leucocyte levels in these groups. This probably reflects differences between the regions in both social class distribution and dietary habits. Social class differences in intake of vitamin C have been known for several years (National Food Survey Committee, Annual Reports, 1970–2; Smithells *et al.*, 1977). These differences are probably associated with income (O'Sullivan *et al.*, 1968) and it is hardly surprising to find them reflected in body reserves of vitamin C.

Seasonal Differences. A number of workers have shown that there are seasonal differences in vitamin C reserves and some of these publications have suggested that the lowest levels in Britain are to be found in winter (Andrews, Brook and Allen, 1966; Bates *et al.*, 1979). These findings apparently agree with the seasonal change in intake of vitamin C (National Food Survey Committee, 1973–6) where the lowest intakes appear to be in the winter quarter. There are, however, reports of equally low or lower vitamin C reserves in the spring (March–May) in Britain (Griffiths, 1968; Milne *et al.*, 1971; Schorah *et al.*, 1978) and low spring values are seen in other European countries (Trier, 1940; Hagtvet, 1945; Ginter, Kajaba and Nizner, 1970). These findings would agree with the observations of Davidson, Passmore and Brock (1972) and Vilter (1967) that scurvy tends to occur most commonly in spring and early summer. Apparent conflict with the National Food Survey Committee (1973–6) could be accounted for by the fact that the spring quarter is an average of the initial low intakes in April and May and the higher ones in June. Indeed the lowest consumption of ascorbic acid in the UK in 1971 occurred in March and April (Buss, D. H., National Food Survey Committee, personal communication). Direct analysis of food has suggested that the lowest intakes in residential accommodation occurred in March and April and at these times intakes were only 60 per cent of the recommended although the yearly average was above the recommended (Harris and Olliver, 1943). In this study, calculated and measured vitamin C intakes were in close agreement, suggesting that cooking practice was especially good. What then are the seasonal changes in those institutions where the preparation of food leads to marked loss of vitamin C (Eddy, 1968)?

If intakes are lowest in the spring, this is likely to occur because of the consumption of the old potato which is low in vitamin C at this time of the year (McCance and Widdowson, 1960). Loss of vitamin C from spring cabbage stored from April to July has been noted by Millross *et al.* (1973) and the general unavailability and expense of fresh fruit and salad materials at this time of the year are likely to contribute to the problem.

There is general agreement that the highest vitamin C reserves are seen in the months of July to October (Milne *et al.*, 1971; Schorah *et al.*, 1978) and these findings are supported by the National Food Survey Committee publications (1973–6) indicating that the highest intakes are in the summer months.

Social class and seasonal differences in vitamin C reserves are thus largely influenced by diet and as Allen, Brook and Broadbent (1968) have pointed out, in combination they can mean that a large proportion of individuals from the lower income groups can fail to reach the recommended intakes at certain times of the year. This is reflected by leucocyte vitamin C reserves in the poor during April and May where levels can be considerably lower than the concentration that is found in the more affluent sections of the population in summer (Schorah *et al.*, 1978).

The Effect of Age on Vitamin C Reserves. It has long been known that both plasma and leucocyte vitamin C concentrations fall with increasing age in both males and females (Kirk and Chieffi, 1953a; Bowers and Kubik, 1965; Kataria and Rao, 1965; Andrews, Brook and Allen, 1966; Brook and Grimshaw, 1968; Bates, Hughes and Hurley, 1972) and age differences persist at different seasons (Trier, 1940). Although the rate of fall decreases in the elderly it still exists within the age range 60–90 years (Milne *et al.*, 1971; Burr *et al.*, 1974). Levels in tissue such as brain and muscle also fall with age (Schaus, 1957; Kirk, 1962) and can fall to as little as 25 per cent of those found in the child (Lewin, 1976), although these tissue assessments have been made at post-mortem and suffer from the problem that in the elderly chronic disease is more likely to precede death with a corresponding decrease in reserves due to the disease process, than in younger individuals who are more likely to have died suddenly from trauma (Willis and Fishman, 1955). As outlined below in the section on institutionalisation, the elderly in hospital have considerably lower levels than the elderly outside institutions, but most of the above studies have shown age changes in those living at home and so institutional cooking has not been a causative factor.

There are reasons to believe that most of the decrease occuring with age is not caused by some metabolic change in the individual but is a result of differences in dietary habits between the young and the elderly. O'Sullivan and co-workers (1968) and Loh (1971) have noted that vitamin C intake decreases in both males and females with increasing age and McClean, Dodds and Stewart (1976), studying a New Zealand population, and Milne and colleagues (1971) in the UK, have found a much higher proportion of elderly males with intakes less than the recommended level than would be found in younger groups (National Food Survey Committee, 1973–6). Intakes in the USA, which appear to be higher than in the UK (Roderuck *et al.*, 1958; Miller *et al.*, 1977; National Food Survey Committee, 1976; Smithells *et al.*, 1977), do not change with age significantly in those living at home and neither does plasma vitamin C (Morgan, Gillum and Williams, 1955; Roderuck *et al.*, 1958). However, Kirk and Chieffi (1953a) using an institutionalised population on a similar diet found an age change in males, but in this study considerably higher levels were noted in the young not on a hospital diet, again indicating the importance of intake. It is just possible that Kirk and Chieffi's findings, made on whole blood, reflect a difference between the effect of age on plasma and leucocyte vitamin C. All the studies where dietary intake has been matched in the different age groups have measured plasma vitamin C. Whilst no age differences are seen in the plasma measurements when intakes are similar, differences could still persist in the leucocyte and Kirk's whole blood measurement would receive up to half its contribution of vitamin C from the leucocyte population. This question will remain unanswered until we have leucocyte measurements in the different age groups matched for intake.

Three studies based on urinary excretion of vitamin C following oral loads (a technique described in Section 2.3.4), have suggested that the elderly may have a higher requirement for vitamin C and these publications are summarised by Irwin and Hutchins (1976). However, it has been pointed out that saturation tests based on a urinary response without the measurement of serum levels, may not be satisfactory in the elderly due to reduced renal function (O'Sullivan *et al.*, 1968; Mitra, 1970). Kirk and Chieffi (1953b) suggest that the rapid fall in whole blood C in the elderly following withdrawal of C supplements indicates an increased metabolic requirement in this age group, but the rate of decrease they report is no more rapid than that found by Hodges and colleagues (1971) in younger individuals depleted of C.

Hence, almost all the evidence currently available points to intake as the main factor influencing age changes in vitamin C reserves. It may be that as we age we eat less and prefer foods that contain little vitamin C. Alternatively, it may be that the present elderly population acquired their dietary habits at a time when vitamin C containing foods were less popular than they have been in recent years. If this latter reason is the case then we shall see the diet of the elderly gradually improve with time; if the former is true then it will remain poor in vitamin C content. It should be noted that age changes are less easily noticed in those individuals who already have depleted vitamin C reserves. In those who smoke (McClean *et al.*, 1976) and those who have low reserves because they are acutely ill (Wilson, 1972) or have been in institutions for long periods of time (Schorah *et al.*, 1981) age changes are either absent or far less marked.

Institutionalisation. The work of Eddy (1968), Disselduff, Murphy and La (1968) and Dawson and Duncan (1975) indicates that the loss of vitamin C during the preparation of food in institutions is considerable, so much so that it is estimated that vitamin C intake of patients in many hospitals is considerably lower than the recommended (Eddy, 1968). These findings are reflected by low vitamin C reserves that have been found in patients living for long periods in hospitals (Morgan, Gillum and Williams, 1955; Kataria and Rao, 1965; Andrews, Brook and Allen, 1966; Schorah *et al.*, 1981). Many of these studies have been on the elderly; age, as indicated in the previous section, could also play a part in precipitating low vitamin C reserves in these groups, but most studies have attempted to take account of this by comparing individuals living at home and in different institutions who are of a similar age. There is also evidence that younger people in institutions have low C levels compared with those of similar age living at home (Dawson and

Table 4.3: Loss of Significant Differences between Vitamin C Reserves in Males and Females at Low Vitamin C Levels

	Vitamin C (Mean Values)	
	$\mu g/10^8$ leucocytes	mg/100 ml plasma
Females	10.7	0.17
Males	8.0	0.17

differences could contribute to a change in vitamin C metabolism. There is evidence to support this. Lower vitamin C reserves are maintained in women who are on oestrogen as opposed to progesterone oral contraceptives (Briggs and Briggs, 1973). However, a final understanding of the differences that exist between males and females with regard to vitamin C metabolism will have to await the application of isotope studies as outlined in Section 2.3.4.

Smoking and Vitamin C Reserves. There is general agreement that smoking lowers the level of vitamin C in both plasma and leucocytes (Brook and Grimshaw, 1968; Pelletier, 1968; Elwood, Hughes and Hurley, 1970; McClean *et al.*, 1976; Keith and Driskell, 1980). Yeung (1976) however finds no difference in women smokers when vitamin C intakes are high. Exton-Smith (1980) was unable to show a difference in the elderly who smoked, and this probably further illustrates that metabolic influences are obscured when body vitamin C reserves are low. The reason for the effect of smoking on vitamin C is unknown. Calder, Curtis and Fore (1963) showed that the effect is not short-term. They were unable to find any decrease in plasma vitamin C in smokers and non-smokers who were asked to smoke very heavily for periods of six hours, but were able to confirm the long-term effect of smoking on both plasma and leucocyte vitamin C concentrations. Poorer intake of vitamin C in smokers than in non-smokers would appear not to play a major part in the difference in reserves between the two groups (Brook and Grimshaw, 1968; Pelletier, 1975). Pelletier's (1975) work shows that smokers with high vitamin C intakes have vitamin C reserves that are no higher than non-smokers whose intakes were less satisfactory.

In early pregnancy both the frequency of poor vitamin C intakes and smoking increase with increasing social class number (Smithells *et al.*, 1977; Schorah *et al.*, 1978). This might suggest that reduced intake is the cause of vitamin C depletion occurring in smokers in this group, because both smoking and intake could be indirectly linked through social class (Section 4.1.1) without implicating any cause and effect relationship. However, smoking lowers vitamin C reserves in each social class grouping (Schorah *et al.*, 1978) suggesting once more that the mechanism is largely independent of dietary intake. It has been suggested that smokers have decreased body reserves of vitamin C as they require more vitamin C orally for their tissues to become saturated. However, when their tissues are saturated they seem to lose vitamin C at the same rate as non-smokers indicating that smokers do not have an increased metabolism, but perhaps a reduced ability to absorb the vitamin (Pelletier, 1968). However, isotope techniques used to study vitamin C utilisation have suggested that there are marked changes in vitamin C metabolism in smokers (Hornig, D., 1981, personal communication).

Although we do not understand the mechanism of the smoking effect on vitamin metabolism, a contributing factor could be the increasing numbers of leucocytes that are seen in those who smoke (Friedman *et al.*, 1973). Correcting for the increase in leucocyte number in smokers shows that the total leucocyte vitamin levels in the blood are far less affected by smoking than the vitamin C content of each leucocyte. In other words, although vitamin C levels fall in the individual leucocyte, the increase in the number of these cells ensures that the total leucocyte vitamin C changes little in the smoker (Schorah *et al.*, 1978).

Racial Differences. Large differences are reported for vitamin C reserves throughout the world with some of the highest values recorded in North America and some of the lowest in India (Morgan, Gillum and Williams, 1955; Roderuck *et al.*, 1958; Ram, 1965). Such differences may be predominantly dietary (Srikantia, Mohanram and Krishnaswamy, 1970), but the reason for including racial differences in this section is illustrated by several publications which suggest that it is very difficult to raise leucocyte vitamin C levels in Indians to those found in Europeans even with intakes of up to 2 g per day (Ram, 1965; Srikantia, Mohanram and Krishnaswamy, 1970; Prasad, 1975; Shilotri and Bhat, 1977). Intakes of this order maintain high plasma concentrations in the Indian (Ram, 1965), so the studies may reflect a difference only in leucocyte metabolism.

Fox and colleagues (1940) reporting on 'native mineworkers' suggest that scurvy develops at intakes which are very much higher than would normally lead to scurvy in the Caucasian. In contrast it is surprising that the nomadic tribes of the southern Sahara, Upper Volta and the northern territories of Nigeria and Ghana do not develop scurvy on a diet almost devoid of fresh fruit and vegetables. Possible synthesis of ascorbic acid by some races might be implicated here, a suggestion for which there is almost no evidence, except an observation that Ghanian children who are malnourished apparently maintain surprisingly high plasma vitamin C concentrations (Neumann *et al.*, 1975). These observations do not prove racial differences, but suggest that we should not automatically accept as a standard for other races findings in Caucasians on whom almost all of the studies in this book have been undertaken.

4.1.3 Summary

There are clearly a number of factors which can affect the vitamin C reserves of the healthy. Some of these, such as social class, regional differences, season, institutionalisation and age, primarily affect intake of the vitamin, although in the latter case an effect on vitamin C metabolism cannot be excluded. Differences due to sex and smoking are clearly due less to dietary change and here we have to look to changes in absorption, metabolism or excretion of the vitamin for an explanation. There is evidence that it is possible to override some differences in metabolism by saturating the body with high intakes (Yeung, 1976), or alternatively some metabolic differences are minimised or are not expressed when vitamin C intakes are so low that body reserves are negligible. Examples of this are the age effect on vitamin C in the institutionalised, particularly during the spring when intakes are poor (Schorah *et al.*, 1981), and the effect of smoking on vitamin C reserves in the unskilled and semi-skilled (Schorah *et al.*, 1978).

Some of these influences on vitamin C reserves exert only a marginal effect. However, in combination their effects can be striking. This is illustrated in a study of early pregnancy where vitamin C reserves were found to be adequate in the majority of women but where a combination of the dietary and metabolic disadvantages of the spring season, smoking and a working-class background combined to produce a small sub-group where vitamin C reserves were far lower than the average found in the whole population (Schorah *et al.*, 1978). It is even more striking in the elderly who are hospitalised for long periods, where a combination of the dietary limitations of institutionalised food preparation, season and old age can ensure very low vitamin C reserves in these patients (Figures 4.3 and 4.4). It is possible that such levels are injurious to health and we shall examine this problem further when

Figure 4.3: Leucocyte Vitamin C Concentrations Found in Various Population Groups in the UK (Mean, 95 per cent Range and Number of Samples). The upper limit for scurvy and the lower limit for the healthy adult are derived from our own studies and reports in the literature (see text).

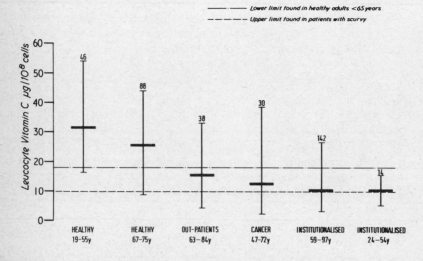

considering what vitamin C reserves are appropriate (Section 4.3).

4.2 The Effect of Disease on Vitamin C Reserves

Evidence that vitamin C reserves are depleted in disease is now over-whelming. The disease can either be acute or chronic and in the former it is surprising how rapidly vitamin C levels fall. We are uncertain whether metabolic change or dietary restriction are primarily respon-sible, but both probably contribute to different extents in different conditions. In acute disease it is unlikely that the changes occurring in plasma and the leucocyte vitamin C can be caused by dietary restriction because of the speed at which they occur. In contrast, in chronic disease, particularly when the condition is advanced, there will often be anorexia and this will greatly contribute to the low vitamin C values found.

It will be clear from the preceding section that many influences, other than state of health, can affect vitamin C reserves. Thus it is important when studying the effects of chronic disease on vitamin C to

Figure 4.4: Plasma Vitamin C Concentrations found in Various Population Groups in the UK (Mean, 95 per cent Range and Number of Samples). The upper limit for scurvy and the lower limit for the healthy adult are derived from our own studies and reports in the literature (see text).

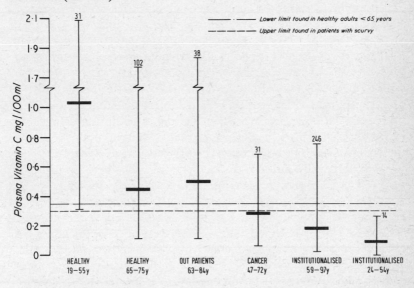

ensure that the non-disease and disease groups are closely matched for age, sex and length of time in hospital and that samples from both groups are collected at the same time of year. If these precautions are observed then any differences found between the groups are more likely to be an effect of the disease process rather than the influence of these other variables. Unfortunately, in the past not all workers have selected their control group with sufficient care and hence it is sometimes difficult to know whether other factors, particularly age and the effect of institutionalisation in long-stay hospitals, are contributing to the difference in vitamin C reserves that have been attributed to the disease process. We shall bear these problems in mind when making an assessment of the evidence in the next two sections.

4.2.1 Acute Disease

In 1937, Faulkner and Taylor commented on the fact that early writers such as Maynwaringe (1672) and Lind (1753) had noted that scurvy often followed an epidemic of infection in a population. Faulkner and Taylor (1937) investigated the effect of infection on vitamin C reserves and found that when people were on an adequate intake serum levels were markedly depressed by acute infection. This, they considered, was unlikely to be due to change in intake as measurements were made within one or two days of the onset of the disease. They were unable to find any effect of infection on vitamin C in those who had initially low vitamin reserves. At about the same time, Rinehart, Greenberg and Christie (1936) reported that rheumatic fever was associated with decreased plasma vitamin C levels in groups matched for age and sex. In pulmonary tuberculosis the decrease in vitamin reserves, as reflected by urine output, was proportional to the activity and severity of the disease. This effect was almost certainly not due to decreased renal function as large differences between the infected and the controls were seen following large oral doses of C and inappropriate urine excretions persisted in the sick even during prolonged periods of high intakes (Abbasy, Harris and Ellman, 1937; Martin and Heise, 1937).

One of the most investigated acute conditions has been the common cold. The effectiveness of high-dose vitamin C treatment in this infection will be assessed in Chapter 5, but here it is relevant to consider the way upper respiratory tract infections may affect the metabolism of vitamin C. Hume and Weyers (1973) have found a significant fall in leucocyte vitamin C during the first days of infection. Considerable quantities of dietary vitamin C (6 g during the first three days of the cold) were required to maintain leucocyte values at the pre-cold level. Davies and colleagues (1979), in a carefully controlled trial, infected subjects with the common cold whilst they were receiving 100 mg of vitamin C per day. During the period of infection urine ascorbic acid and diketogluconic acid fell compared with the controls and this was considered to reflect increased metabolism of the vitamin. Plasma and urine levels also fell during an experimentally-induced cold infection in another study (Schwartz *et al.*, 1973). In spite of one publication which showed no effect of acute sand-fly disease on vitamin C levels (Beisel *et al.*, 1972), the evidence is now in favour of some change in the metabolism of the vitamin during acute infection.

Not only does infection influence vitamin C levels but other acute forms of trauma are capable of lowering vitamin C levels in the blood. Concentrations of vitamin C have been shown to fall within a few hours of onset of chest pain in myocardial infarction and they remained depressed for up to two weeks following the attack (Hume *et al.*, 1972; Machtey, Syrkis and Fried, 1975). Plasma and leucocyte vitamin C levels have also been found to drop rapidly following surgery, falling to as low as 50 per cent of the original value (Lund, 1939; Bartlett, Jones and Ryan, 1940; Irvin, Chattopadhyay and Smythe, 1978). Concentrations return to normal within seven days of surgery providing neither transfusion nor sepsis complicates the post-operative course (McGinn and Hamilton, 1976; Hill *et al.*, 1977). In order to prevent this post-surgical decline considerable quantities of vitamin C, of the order of 300–500 mg/day, are required (Crandon *et al.*, 1958; Shukla, 1969). In contrast burns are not associated with a decreased leucocyte vitamin C although there is evidence that burned skin accumulates vitamin C in comparison to surrounding normal skin, suggesting a need for the vitamin in the repair process (Barton, Laing and Barisoni, 1972).

The reason for such a marked change in metabolism during acute trauma and disease is completely unknown. It is possible that some of the changes seen reflect a redistribution of the vitamin C between different cellular and fluid compartments in the body. For example, the increase in leucocyte number which accompanies acute infection could lower the concentration per leucocyte because the newly released cells could either contain less vitamin C (Vallance, Hume and Weyers, 1978) or they could artificially dilute the platelet contribution to the leucocyte measurement as described in Section 2.3.3 and shown experimentally by Evans, Currie and Campbell (1980). However, the lack of evidence for an increase in urine excretion of the vitamin (Bartlett, Jones and Ryan, 1940; Shukla, 1969) and the decreases in plasma levels during acute conditions would seem to confirm that some fundamental change in vitamin C metabolism is occurring. Increased oxidation of vitamin C is suggested by work indicating a considerable increase in plasma dehydroascorbic acid during acute illness, the levels becoming very high in those who subsequently die from their condition (Charkrabarti and Banerjee, 1955). It has been suggested, however, that it is difficult to measure dehydroascorbic acid concentrations accurately using current techniques (Chapter 2).

4.2.2 Chronic Disease

Faulkner and Taylor (1937), in their study of acute infection, also noted that four patients with chronic disease had low vitamin C concentrations and required up to 200–300 mg/day in order to bring their reserves into the normal range. Since then, low vitamin C reserves have been noted in association with a number of other conditions particularly gastrointestinal disease (Ingalls and Warren, 1937; Portnoy and Wilkinson, 1938; Booth and Todd, 1972; Hughes and Williams, 1978; Linaker, 1979), liver disease, especially alcoholic liver disease (Beattie and Sherlock, 1976; BMJ, 1977; Bonjour, 1979), alcoholism

(Lester, Buccino and Bizzocco, 1960; Sviripa, 1971; O'Keane, Russell and Goldberg, 1972) and asthma (Olusi *et al.*, 1979). The overall effect of chronic disease on depleting vitamin reserves has been summarised by Kelleher (1979).

One condition which is of particular interest is diabetes. There is evidence from animal work that the ability of insulin to decrease blood glucose levels can be enhanced by high-dose vitamin C (Losert, Vetter and Wendt, 1980). In the human it has been noted that low vitamin C levels produce a diabetic type of glucose tolerance curve and that repletion of vitamin C with large oral intakes reduces insulin require- ments for the diabetic (Dice and Daniel, 1973). Ginter and colleagues (1978) have noted that vitamin C is lower in the plasma and leucocytes of diabetics, age and sex matched with controls. They suggest that this may be due to an inability to transport vitamin C into the cells as the leucocyte levels were proportionally lower than the plasma concentra- tion. The transport of vitamin C across the cell wall is believed to be in the form of dehydroascorbic acid which is less ionised than ascorbic acid at physiological pH and is therefore more membrane permeable. This transport may be inhibited by glucose (Mann and Newton, 1975) and this may explain why cell vitamin C concentrations are reduced and plasma dehydroascorbic acid concentrations are higher (Chatterjee *et al.*, 1975) in the diabetic where blood glucose concentrations are high. Low-platelet C may enhance the aggregation of platelets and thus have important implications for the health of the diabetic (Sarji, Kleinfelder and Brewington, 1979). It has also been suggested that, as vitamin C is implicated in collagen synthesis (Section 3.1.1), these low cellular levels of the vitamin may be connected with microvascular connective tissue changes which occur in the diabetic and are believed to be responsible for the organ damage seen in the condition (Mann and Newton, 1975).

Pregnancy is another chronic condition which affects vitamin C reserves. There are a number of studies which indicate that plasma vitamin C concentrations decrease gradually throughout pregnancy (Vobecky *et al.*, 1974; Rivers and Devine, 1975). Leucocyte levels also appear to decrease, but pregnancy, as acute disease, is associated with an increased number of leucocytes and it has been shown that total circulating leucocyte vitamin C is changed little during pregnancy, although the concentration within each leucocyte is reduced (Schorah *et al.*, 1978). Human milk contains high concentrations of vitamin C and so lactation can potentially lead to significant losses of maternal vitamin C, of the order of 32 mg/day (Woodruff, 1964). This loss could account for the low vitamin C levels that have been found in lactating women (Martin *et al.*, 1957).

There is no doubt that chronic disease is often accompanied by a decreased dietary intake (Ingalls and Warren, 1937). Finkle (1937) believed that most of the decreased excretion he found in hospital patients was due to decreased intake. It is probable, therefore, that some of the decrease in plasma and leucocyte vitamin C in chronic disease must reflect a decreased dietary intake. Chronic disease is also more frequent in the elderly and therefore the age effect considered in Section 4.1.1 could also play its part in decreasing ascorbic acid reserves, again largely through reduced intake. Finally, there is the problem that some individuals suffering from chronic disease have been in hospital for long periods. However, in most studies this has probably not been a complicating factor. Indeed, a number of workers have attempted to account for these problems by using age- and sex-matched controls to compare with their disease populations (Olusi *et al.*, 1979; Hughes and Williams, 1978) or even matched for dietary intake (Linaker, 1979). Whilst such matching for intake may be possible in gastrointestinal disease, it is far more difficult in liver disease where dietary intakes are often reduced and may explain most of the vitamin C depletion in this condition (Leevy, Thompson and Baker, 1970). This is particularly so with regard to alcoholic liver disease and this has been stressed by Bonjour (1979). Alcoholics without any obvious liver disease also appear to decrease their ascorbic acid intakes (O'Keane, Russell and Goldberg, 1972). Bonjour (1979) however, considers that although low intakes are partially responsible for reduced vitamin C levels, there is possibly a direct effect of alcohol consumption. This is supported by the large daily intakes that appear to be required in alcoholic liver disease in order to maintain vitamin C excretion within the normal range (Sviripa, 1971). In addition in non-alcoholic liver disease, marked deficiency could not be accounted for entirely by decreased intake (Morgan *et al.*, 1976).

4.2.3 Summary

Are low vitamin C reserves in disease primarily caused by poor dietary intake, as in part for chronic disease, or by a change in metabolism, as would seem to be the overriding feature of an acute condition? The answer will have to await studies which can examine vitamin C metabolism in more detail using the isotopic techniques of Kallner, Hartmann and Hornig (1979) and Baker and colleagues (1971). Whatever the reason, reduced C reserves are found in most people who are ill. One could argue that rather than needing lower reserves, these individuals may require a higher level of vitamin C than the healthy in order to facilitate drug metabolism and wound healing and supply the general increase in metabolism caused by infection or trauma. It would therefore be appropriate to examine the need for vitamin C in both health and disease and try to assess whether reserves that are found in these groups are adequate or not.

4.3 Appropriate Vitamin C Reserves in Man

In preceding sections of this book, we have been able to draw some conclusions about vitamin C. But we now come to an area about which there is considerable controversy and little clear-cut evidence. The confusion is typified by the recommended dietary allowances for the USA, which have changed no less than three times during the last twelve years, values for the adult decreasing from 70 to 45 mg in 1974 (Young, 1964; Food and Nutrition Board, 1974) and rising to 60 mg in 1980 (Food and Nutrition Board, 1980). There are different recommendations from country to country, the UK being one of the lowest at 30 mg per day (Department of Health and Social Security, 1969). Such differences are in part due to what the recommendations of different countries reflect; those in the USA are adequate to meet the needs of practically all healthy persons, whilst those in the UK refer to a representative individual in the population so that some will require more, others less (Young, 1964). They also reflect limitations in the way dietary recommendations are estimated. Dietary recommendations are assessed from an extrapolation of the requirements of animals, a knowledge of the dietary intake found in healthy humans and the findings of the few studies on humans who have been depleted experimentally. For vitamin C, the first two procedures are unsatisfactory. There are few mammals that are dependent on a dietary source of vitamin C (Chapter 1). Because of availability and low cost, most experimental work has been done with the guinea pig, although this animal metabolises vitamin C in a manner which differs from the human, having a more rapid turnover and converting most of the vitamin to CO_2 (Woodruff, 1964; Chapter 1).

An attempt to assess recommended intakes from diets found in 'healthy' individuals can also be argued as invalid. There is believed to be considerable biological variation in the human, some individuals requiring apparently very little vitamin C to prevent scurvy, others considerably more (Yew, 1975). In addition, vitamin C has been implicated in the aetiology of some of the major degenerative diseases (Chapters 3 and 5). The frequency in the general population of some of these diseases (e.g. cancer and arterial disease) makes it certain that within a so-called healthy group many individuals will be developing these conditions. If lack of vitamin C encourages the development of these diseases, it would clearly be useless to use vitamin C intakes in this so-called healthy population as a reference range for adequate intake, as these values could be encouraging the development of these major diseases. Whilst it must be emphasised that there is, as yet, insufficient evidence for us to be convinced that vitamin C depletion is implicated in these conditions, there is sufficient circumstantial evidence to question whether we can assume that vitamin C intakes in the apparently healthy are adequate for all our needs. Hence, the only reference point that has been acceptably assessed is the intake required to prevent the symptoms of clinical scurvy in individuals who have been artificially depleted of the vitamin (Crandon, Lund and Dill, 1940; Bartley, Krebs and O'Brien, 1953; Hodges *et al.*, 1971).

Publications using these procedures have produced remarkably consistent results, suggesting that healthy young men require intakes of the order of 10 mg or rather less per day to treat and prevent the development of the symptoms of scurvy. Here then is our corner-stone, the one piece of solid undisputed evidence about C requirements. When blood levels have been measured in these studies, some have indicated that plasma and leucocyte vitamin C concentrations are effectively zero when signs of clinical scurvy are seen (Crandon, Lund and Dill, 1940; Bartley, Krebs and O'Brien, 1953). However, others, during both experimental depletion and clinical practice, have found that blood vitamin C values are measurable when the signs of scurvy are present (Goldberg, 1963; Walker, 1968; Hodges *et al.*, 1971; Exton-Smith, 1980). We have also found measurable vitamin C reserves in cases of scurvy and the mean values for our scorbutic group have been shown in Figure 4.1. Overall, these results and those of other workers suggest that vitamin C concentrations in patients with scurvy fall within the ranges 0.0 to 10.0 μg per 10^8 leucocytes and 0.0 to 0.3 mg per 100 ml plasma. The upper limits of these ranges are presented in Figures 4.3 and 4.4 along with examples of mean values and ranges for vitamin C reserves found in a number of populations we have studied. It is clear that some individuals have vitamin C reserves that fall within the range where clinical scurvy is seen and in some groups this can be as high as 50 per cent of the population (Table 4.4). The proportions in Table 4.4 are taken from the leucocyte

Table 4.4: Proportion of Population Groups Who Have Leucocyte Vitamin C Concentrations Below the Upper Limits Found in Hypovitaminosis C (A) and Clinical Scurvy (B)

Group	A[a]	B[b]
Young healthy	3	0
Elderly healthy	20	3
Elderly out-patients	68	20
Patients with cancer	76	46
Institutionalised elderly	95	50
Institutionalised young	100	30

Notes: a. Proportion (%) with leucocyte vitamin C values less than 95 per cent range found in young healthy subjects and equivalent to those found in hypovitaminosis C. b. Proportion (%) with leucocyte vitamin C equivalent to those found in scurvy.

measurements rather than the plasma, because the upper limit for plasma vitamin C in scurvy reported in the literature (0.3 mg/100 ml) is higher, rather than lower, than that which would be maintained by a 10 mg/day intake which would prevent the disease (Figure 4.6). Such high plasma values probably reflect a transient elevation, possibly due to a slight improvement in vitamin C intake at the time of presentation. Such a change would not affect leucocyte levels. Indeed intakes of 10 mg/d maintain 95 per cent of individuals above 9 $\mu g/10^8$ leucocytes (Figure 4.5) which fits very closely to the suggested threshold at which clinical scurvy can develop, 10 $\mu g/10^8$ cells.

Although the majority of subjects having leucocyte levels less than this threshold do not have scurvy, a high incidence of the disease may only be avoided in these at-risk individuals by the increased intake of the vitamin which occurs in late May and lasts till October (Section 4.1.1, seasonal differences). This increase probably lifts vitamin C reserves above the levels associated with clinical scurvy and found in winter and spring (the concentrations illustrated in Figures 4.3 and 4.4 were measured at this time) just in time to prevent the development of overt scurvy in a large number of these individuals. However, in spite of this the incidence of the disease is surprisingly high in those groups where the frequency of low levels is highest; the sick, the institutionalised and the elderly (Milner, 1963; Mitra, 1970; Exton-Smith, 1980). Because of this and because of the insidious onset of the condition and the lack of specificity of the early clinical signs which include behavioural changes, weakness, lethargy and skin lesions, it would seem to be against sensible health-care practice to allow an individual

Figure 4.5: The Relationship between Leucocyte Vitamin C Levels and Intake of the Vitamin. The shaded area represents the 95 per cent range for mean values in reports published during the last 40 years.

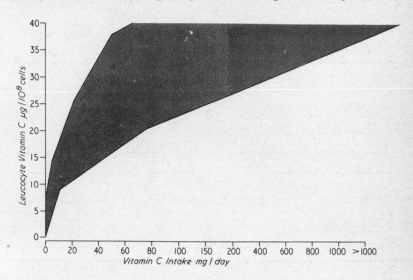

to have vitamin C levels below this threshold. There is additional cause for concern because many who do so are in hospital and, as argued earlier, they may require higher reserves because the vitamin is being utilised more rapidly. The fact that such low levels occur in hospitals emphasises the inadequacy of food preparation in many institutions.

A minimum intake of 10 mg per day with leucocyte levels of at least 10 μg per 10^8 cells may seem sufficient, as these reserves will certainly prevent scurvy in the majority of subjects. The problem with this argument is that recognised symptoms of acute scurvy may not be the only changes which result from vitamin C depletion; other diseases, encouraged by low vitamin C levels, may develop over many years in people with higher vitamin C reserves and intakes than patients with clinical scurvy. There is evidence that in the guinea pig there are two conditions: acute clinical scurvy which will develop in this animal in 15–20 days on a vitamin C free diet, and chronic sub-clinical vitamin C deficiency (hypovitaminosis C) which develops over a period of months on higher intakes of the vitamin and presents with clinical, physiological and biochemical features which are different from those of acute scurvy (Sulkin and Sulkin, 1975; Ginter, 1979a).

Does hypovitaminosis C cause disease and degenerative change in the

84   *Vitamin C in Health and Disease*

Figure 4.6: The Relationship between Plasma Vitamin C Levels and Intake of the Vitamin. The shaded area represents the 95 per cent range for the mean values in reports published during the last 40 years.

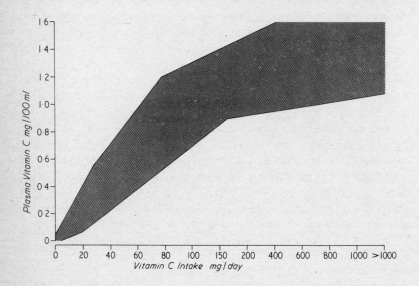

human? If it does, what intakes and tissue reserves of the vitamin will be preventive? We now step from our corner-stone of 10 mg per day, the intake known to prevent acute scurvy, on to shifting sand, for there are no clear answers to these questions, but a summary of the evidence will serve to provide provisional recommendations.

4.3.1 Changes Associated with Hypovitaminosis C

We must begin with a definition of hypovitaminosis C and also emphasise the difference between association and cause. The evidence from the first section of this chapter clearly indicates that a very wide range of plasma and leucocyte vitamin C concentrations can be found in subjects living in developed nations. It may be argued that, as some of the degenerative change which is associated with hypovitaminosis C grows out of this population, almost all levels represent hypovitaminosis C. This is a difficult hypothesis to test and, on the assumption that the lowest levels should be associated with the greatest risk, we will define hypovitaminosis C as a plasma or leucocyte level less than the lower limits of the 95 per cent range of healthy adults younger than 65 years of age. Several publications and our own data suggest lower limits for this population of between 0.2 to 0.5 mg per 100 ml of plasma and 15 to 21 μg per 10^8 leucocytes (Denson and Bowers, 1961; Sauberlich, 1975; Schorah *et al.*, 1978; Schorah, 1979; Exton-Smith, 1980). For the purpose of this discussion we will average these lower limits and assume hypovitaminosis C occurs in the absence of clinical scurvy at plasma levels less than 0.35 mg per 100 ml and leucocyte concentrations less than 18 μg per 10^8 cells. Reference to Figures 4.3 and 4.4 where these limits are marked and Table 4.4 shows that approximately 20 per cent of the 'healthy' elderly adult population of the UK fall below these limits and that this proportion increases as chronic disease and/or institutionalisation further deplete body vitamin C reserves. Indeed, the majority of patients in hospital for long periods have values below these limits.

Although chronic disease and general deterioration in health are associated with vitamin C reserves below this threshold, association does not necessarily mean cause and effect. It is possible for two independent factors to be related through a third without directly affecting each other. A simple example would be the higher death rate found in hospitals compared with outside. An external observer who knew nothing about this world might assume that the hospital environment was dangerous and led directly to the increased death rate. Of course this assumption is erroneous as the two factors, mortality and hospitalisation, are indirectly linked to each other through the disease process which increases both the likelihood of admission to hospital and mortality independently. The other point of difficulty when considering cause and effect is deciding which factor is causative and which is affected. Does a clinical condition lead to a low vitamin C value or, alternatively, does the low vitamin C predispose the individual to the condition. The only satisfactory way of solving these problems is to give vitamin C along with a blank (placebo) preparation in an adequately controlled double-blind trial, to see if symptoms believed to be associated with vitamin C depletion are alleviated or prevented. In many published studies such trials have either not been undertaken or have been inadequate to draw satisfactory conclusions. Hence a publication reporting an association between a clinical condition and low vitamin C does not prove that the vitamin causes the condition. Alternatively, because the degenerative changes that could result from hypovitaminosis C, such as arterial degeneration, behavioural change and microaneurisms of small blood vessels, may take many years of hypovitaminosis C to develop and once present may be irreversible, a negative finding from a short-term vitamin C/placebo supplementation trial does not mean that the vitamin has no effect. However, studies that have been undertaken, although limited, can provide some useful information and we shall examine the evidence from such reports to assess the probability that the health of individuals with hypovitaminosis C is affected in a number of ways directly by the poor C reserves.

Behavioural Changes. Changes in mental function are often associated with clinical scurvy (Cutforth, 1958; Walker, 1968). The work of Kinsman and Hood (1971), who observed behavioural changes during artificial vitamin C depletion, suggested that this was one of the early signs of scurvy, and would occur at plasma levels as high as 0.3 to 0.4 mg per 100 ml. Low vitamin C reserves have also been associated with psychiatric diseases such as schizophrenia and depression (Vanderkamp, 1966) and in one study (Milner, 1963) clear improvement in the mental condition has been reported on supplementing subjects with the vitamin. A probable role of vitamin C in the metabolism of neurotransmitters has been described in Section 3.1.1, but we have no information about plasma levels or intakes that are required to maintain this metabolic process adequately. There is, therefore, evidence that vitamin C is required for adequate mental function and that plasma concentrations required to maintain this function are rather higher than those required to prevent scurvy (greater than 0.4 mg per 100 ml).

Increases in plasma vitamin C in animals from 0.1 to 1 mg per 100 ml increase brain vitamin C concentrations by about 75 per cent, but a further quadrupling of the plasma concentration only increases brain vitamin C another 25 per cent. Whilst one might argue that plasma levels of 1 mg per 100 ml should be maintained, because these would produce slightly higher brain concentrations than 0.4 mg per 100 ml, the threshold at which behavioural changes occur (Kinsman and Hood, 1971), there is as yet no evidence that this brings about any physiological advantage to the individual.

Lassitude and Fatigue. Lassitude and fatigue, like behavioural changes, are early clinical manifestations of scurvy. Such changes can be linked to one of the fundamental roles of vitamin C in the synthesis of carnitine, a molecule responsible for carrying fatty acids into the cells' mitochondria and therefore important in energy production (Section 3.1.1). The levels of plasma and leucocyte vitamin C that have been reported to be associated with a decreased ability to work are at the upper limit of concentrations found in clinical scurvy, for example, 0.05 to 0.22 mg per 100 ml (Kinsman and Hood, 1971) and 4–7 μg per

10^8 leucocytes (Crandon, Lund and Dill, 1940; Pijoan and Lozner, 1944).

Wound Healing. Advanced clinical scurvy is associated with poor wound healing and the breakdown of old scar tissue (Anson, 1748; Crandon, Lund and Dill, 1940; Bartley, Krebs and O'Brien, 1953) and vitamin C is known to accumulate in wounds during healing (Bartlett, Jones and Ryan, 1942; Gould, 1963; Barton, Laing and Barisoni, 1972). In experimental studies it is clear that the degree of depletion of vitamin C which must occur before wounds fail to heal is considerable (Crandon, Lund and Dill, 1940; Bartley, Krebs and O'Brien, 1953). In clinical studies, however, wound healing sometimes seems to be affected in the absence of clinical scurvy (Crandon *et al.*, 1961; Gerson, 1975). It is possible that the difference between the experimental and clinical condition reflects a depletion in other vitamins in addition to vitamin C and that these multiple depletions aggravate vitamin C deficiency. We must therefore conclude that only those levels found in clinical scurvy will be inadequate to maintain appropriate wound healing unless there are multiple vitamin deficiencies which may result from chronic disease. In these cases, repletion of other vitamin reserves may also be required for vitamin C to be effective. There is, however, the possibility that certain types of wound may require larger reserves of vitamin C in order to heal effectively. In a double-blind trial of vitamin C in subjects with pressure sores there was a significant improvement in those receiving large doses of vitamin compared with a placebo group (Taylor *et al.*, 1974).

Haemorrhages and Microvaricosities of Small Blood Vessels. These lesions, which occur on the skin and under the tongue and in some cases possibly in organs such as the brain and kidney, would seem to be associated with vitamin C depletion (Bourne, 1938; Taylor, 1966, 1976; Hodges *et al.*, 1971; Irwin and Hutchins, 1976; Exton-Smith, 1980), and do occur in scurvy (Eddy and Taylor, 1977). Attempts to bring about regression of these lesions with vitamin C therapy have largely been unsuccessful (Arthur *et al.*, 1967; Disselduff, Murphy and La, 1968; Andrews, Letcher and Brook, 1969) although we have found some marginal changes in purpura and petechial haemorrhages after two months of vitamin C therapy in the elderly (Schorah *et al.*, 1981). The failure of C to improve markedly these lesions and the fact that they are nearly always found in the elderly may imply that vitamin C depletion makes no direct contribution to their causation, but rather that both vitamin C depletion and the small blood vessel lesions are indirectly associated through ageing. However, there is evidence that the artificial induction of such lesions by increasing capillary pressure with restriction of the flow of venous blood from the arm, are more easily achieved when vitamin C levels are low (Bourne, 1938; Eddy, 1972). There is also good theoretical evidence to implicate vitamin C, as these lesions could be caused by an underlying weakness of the wall of the blood vessel which could have arisen through the changes in connective tissue metabolism which will be present in vitamin C depletion (Section 3.1.1; Eddy and Taylor, 1977). This may mean that the lesions are, in part, caused by vitamin C deficiency but once produced are largely irreversible and would therefore not be expected to respond to large doses of vitamin C given for relatively short periods of time (Eddy and Taylor, 1977).

Because small blood vessel haemorrhages and varicosities may cause serious damage if they occur within the walls of larger blood vessels or within organs such as the brain and kidney (Taylor, 1976; Clemetson, 1979) and because they appear to be irreversible, we would argue that chronically it is necessary to keep body vitamin C reserves higher than the concentrations which are found in subjects who manifest these signs. Eddy (1972) has suggested that changes in capillary fragility are associated with a critical level of leucocyte vitamin C of less than 15 μg per 10^8 cells. Many of the elderly in whom these lesions are found have vitamin C levels less than this with plasma levels less than 0.35 mg/100 ml (Schorah *et al.*, 1979, 1981). These values fit fairly closely to our provisional threshold for hypovitaminosis C (less than 0.35 mg/100 ml plasma or 18 μg/10^8 leucocytes) and hence it would seem appropriate that body reserves should not be allowed to fall below these concentrations for extended periods. There would seem to be no evidence to suggest that short-term depletion below these concentrations, say of no more than two weeks duration, would have any detrimental effects in healthy individuals.

Drug Metabolism. The association of vitamin C depletion with decreased rates of drug metabolism (Section 3.2.1) suggests that patients who are receiving drug therapy should not have low reserves of the vitamin. In liver disease it has been suggested by Beattie and Sherlock (1976) that levels of leucocyte vitamin C of less than 17.5 μg per 10^8 cells are associated with decreased rates of drug metabolism. Again the threshold that we arbitrarily selected for hypovitaminosis C would appear to be the one above which vitamin C reserves should be maintained in those who are on long-term drug therapy in order to prevent possible toxic drug accumulation. This may be particularly crucial in liver disease where drug metabolism may be further reduced by the disease itself.

General Health. In this section on appropriate vitamin C reserves, we have considered conditions not only which are associated with hypo-vitaminosis C but also where the underlying lesion can be explained by a failure of a metabolic process which is associated with one of the biochemical roles of the vitamin outlined in Chapter 3. This final section however deals with general health and therefore is more diffuse and changes described often bear no close association to the known function of the vitamin.

There are a considerable number of publications which have linked vitamin C depletion with deterioration in general health in animals. The work of Ginter (1978, 1979a) has emphasised that moderate vitamin C deficiency in guinea pigs is capable of bringing about many changes which may lead to a gradual deterioration in the health of the animal: for instance increasing blood and tissue cholesterol, changes in the structure of the liver and of the walls of arteries. There is also evidence that intakes of vitamin C above the minimum required to prevent scurvy have a part to play in maintenance of adequate growth and health in the guinea pig (Goldsmith, 1961; Pye, Taylor and Fontanares, 1961; Rivers and Devine, 1975; Veen-Baigent *et al.*, 1975).

There are similar studies in the human. Bates and colleagues (1979) have noted a slow steady weight loss in all elderly subjects where vitamin C was low. Vitamin C supplementation has brought about an increased growth compared with a placebo group in Nigerian children (Nicol, 1956) and in young Americans (Miller *et al.*, 1977) and slight weight gains and increases in plasma proteins have been noted in elderly subjects given vitamin C compared with those receiving placebo supplements (Schorah *et al.*, 1979, 1981). Mothers giving birth to lighter children have a higher incidence of leucocyte vitamin C levels less than 20 μg per 10^8 leucocyte than mothers giving birth to heavier children and this difference could not be accounted for by social class variations which might independently have produced an association between lighter children and low C reserves (Schorah *et al.*, 1978). However, there is little evidence that marginally low vitamin C reserves have any other deleterious effects on the outcome of pregnancy (Vobecky *et al.*, 1974; Rivers and Devine, 1975; Schorah *et al.*, 1978).

Several studies have indicated that, especially in acute disease in the elderly, very low vitamin C levels are associated with an increased mortality (Chope, 1954; Charkrabarti and Banerjee, 1955; Wilson, 1972). Wilson and co-workers (1973) subsequently showed that vitamin C supplementation in these individuals was unable to reduce mortality, although they indicated that in some of these patients it was extremely difficult to elevate vitamin C concentrations even with high oral doses. However, vitamin C therapy has been reported to have been effective in decreasing general illness in younger subjects compared with a control group receiving quinine (Scheunert, 1949). We have also found some general improvement in the elderly in terms of mobility and awareness (Schorah *et al.*, 1978) although we have not been able to confirm this (Schorah *et al.*, 1981).

Large doses of vitamin C (greater than 400 mg/day) have been reported to be effective in preventing or treating a number of diseases including arterial disease, immune deficiency, cancer, upper respiratory tract infection (the common cold) and asthma. Although high-dose vitamin C and not merely correction of hypovitaminosis C has been advocated in these conditions, such high doses may not be needed. Correction of hypovitaminosis C alone may be sufficient or vitamin C may be of little benefit in these conditions. However, the benefits or otherwise of megadose vitamin C therapy in disease will be considered in Chapter 5.

4.3.2 Conclusions

Clearly in man vitamin C reserves should not be allowed to fall to those which are seen in clinical scurvy at any time, especially as some of the earlier clinical signs such as behavioural changes, muscle weakness and lethargy can develop when leucocyte and plasma vitamin C levels are at the upper limit of those seen in scurvy. An argument could be made that reserves should be maintained rather higher than these because of effects on the integrity of small blood vessels, drug metabolism and general health, including decreases in body weight and immune function. The definition of hypovitaminosis C suggested at the beginning of this section would appear to be a provisional working lower limit for vitamin C reserves in those who are healthy. It may not matter that levels fall briefly below this threshold, but they should not persist at these concentrations for longer than a few weeks. There are, however, many individuals who fall below this limit and even a proportion whose reserves are below the scurvy threshold (Figures 4.3 and 4.4; Table 4.4). There is greater cause for concern here, because an increasing frequency of inappropriate values is found in the sick who arguably require more vitamin C rather than less in order to facilitate drug metabolism and wound healing and supply an increased metabolism.

If we are to maintain vitamin C concentrations in individuals above the threshold of hypovitaminosis C, 0.35 mg/100 ml of plasma and 18 μg/10^8 leucocytes, then we must consider what intakes we require to achieve this. Figures 4.5 and 4.6 show the relationship between mean dietary intake and leucocyte and plasma vitamin C respectively for a number of publications plotted as the 95 per cent range of the values. Criteria for inclusion are that subjects should have been on the intake for at least 30 days to allow plasma and leucocyte levels to stabilise to the intake. Only studies in developed countries are included. There is a fairly close relationship between intake and the blood measurements and both the 18 μg and 0.35 mg lower limits for leucocyte and plasma reserves suggest an intake of about 60 mg of the vitamin per day in order to guarantee that 95 per cent of individuals will have a blood concentration above these limits. This intake is not too different from the suggested daily rates for the metabolism of the vitamin (Hodges *et al.*, 1971; Kallner, Hartmann and Hornig, 1979). It is the same as the recommended intake for the USA, but higher than that in the UK although this latter recommendation refers to a representative individual in the population rather than the intake required to guarantee 95 per cent of the population above a threshold. However, it is clear that many households will have intakes lower than even the UK recommended (Allen, Brook and Broadbent, 1968; Exton-Smith, 1980) and the proportion with inadequate intakes is even greater in hospitals and institutions where the intake of most will be below 30 mg/day (Eddy, 1968). We would admit that our suggestion for an intake of 60 mg/day is based on evidence which is still not conclusive, but there would seem to be no excuse now for not maintaining those in hospital on intakes that at least reach the UK recommended level of 30 mg/day. Our suggestion of 60 mg/day will not achieve body saturation in most subjects. For this, consumption of vitamin C should be of the order of 100 mg/day (Irwin and Hutchins, 1976; Kallner, Hartmann and Hornig, 1979), but there is as yet little evidence that tissue saturation will improve our health over and above reserves maintained by 60 mg/day. We also emphasise that the intake is a recommendation for the healthy. It may be that considerably more vitamin C will be required by those who are sick, especially if they are acutely ill. The next chapter will consider whether large doses of vitamin C are of benefit in diseases such as cancer, arterial disease and respiratory tract conditions such as asthma and the common cold.

Finally, it is important to remember that depletion of other vitamins can occur in association with low levels of vitamin C (Leevy, Thompson and Baker, 1970; Mitra, 1970; Nobile, 1974; Woodhill *et al.*, 1974; Morgan *et al.*, 1976; Maclean, Dodds and Stewart, 1976; Vir and Love, 1979; Brin, 1980). This may encourage clinical signs of scurvy to develop at higher vitamin C reserves than are found in scurvy induced experimentally in the human where other vitamin concentrations are adequate. In individuals where vitamin C supplementation is judged to be required, it would therefore be more appropriate to supplement these individuals with multi-vitamin preparations rather than just vitamin C and in trials where this has been undertaken it would seem that the improvements in health of the individuals have been far greater than those that have been found with C supplementation alone (Brocklehurst *et al.*, 1968). An example of this is the possibility that maternal multi-vitamin supplementation can lead to a significant decrease in the incidence of malformations of the neural tube (spina bifida and anencephaly) which may be induced in the fetus by the combined effect of a marginal depletion of several vitamins including vitamin C (Smithells, Sheppard and Schorah, 1976; Smithells *et al.*, 1980).

5 THERAPEUTIC ASPECTS OF VITAMIN C

In recent years several metabolic roles for vitamin C have been suggested (Chapter 3). Some of these roles are such that it is possible to speculate that an enhancement of their functions, which might be encouraged by the vitamin in large doses (10—1,000 times the physiological dose), could have certain prophylactic and therapeutic effects in many pathological conditions. These conditions include infectious diseases, immune deficiency disorders, atherosclerosis, malignant disease, bone pain, tissue healing, mental conditions and allergy. The usefulness of large doses of vitamin C in treating or preventing these diseases, however, is exceedingly controversial.

5.1 Infectious Diseases

The most widely known use of large amounts of vitamin C is for the prevention or relief of symptoms of the common cold. Pauling (1970) suggests that there is an optimum intake of the vitamin and that this may vary with the individual. He advocates the daily ingestion of 1 or 2 g of vitamin C increasing to 4—10 g per day at the onset of cold. According to Pauling such therapy is definitely effective in the prevention and/or amelioration of the common cold, influenza and other infections.

Pauling's suggestions have led to considerable scientific effort to unravel the role of the vitamin in respiratory infections. As outlined in Section 4.2.1, there are indications for a change in the metabolism of the vitamin in the common cold, with rapid loss of the vitamin C from the leucocyte during the early stages of the infection (Hume and Weyers, 1973) and a decrease in plasma and urine vitamin C during experimentally induced infections (Schwartz *et al.*, 1973; Davies *et al.*, 1979). The need for very high intakes to maintain the concentration of vitamin C in leucocytes during infection (Hume and Weyers, 1973) provides scientific support for Pauling's suggestions that C may be beneficial. It is also true that vitamin C may be involved in the body's protective immunological mechanisms (Section 3.2.6) and this could implicate C in a preventive role in infectious disease.

The final proof, however, must come from the success or otherwise of the vitamin in treating or preventing colds in appropriately controlled trials. A number of these have been reported in the last 15 years. Intakes in the trials have ranged from prophylactic doses of 80 mg to 2 g per day, and a dose of up to 8 g per day has been used therapeutically at the onset of cold symptoms. Together, these trials have indicated that such therapy has almost no effect on either the frequency or length of the cold. There are, however, clear indications that the severity of symptoms are decreased by vitamin C treatment in such experiments (Anderson, Reid and Beaton, 1972; Anderson *et al.*, 1975; Coulehan *et al.*, 1974; Miller *et al.*, 1977; Baird *et al.*, 1979; Pitt and Costrin, 1979). In some trials the improvement has led to an actual decrease in the number of days of disability as assessed by days away from work (Anderson, Reid and Beaton, 1972; Anderson *et al.*, 1975). Not only are symptoms less severe, but there is the suggestion that complications such as pneumonia are less likely to develop in those on high-dose therapy (Pitt and Costrin, 1979). Both Chalmers (1975) and Coulehan (1979) in their reviews on the efficacy of vitamin C in the common cold acknowledge that there is a decrease in the severity of the symptoms, although Chalmers attaches more significance to this than does Coulehan. One underlying factor which is typical of many of the trials where vitamin C reserves have been measured is that the initial plasma concentrations of vitamin C are often very good, in the order of 1 mg/100 ml or greater (Anderson, 1977; Miller *et al.*, 1977; Pitt and Costrin, 1979). These reserves approach the level of tissue saturation and an increase in vitamin C intake only brings about a small increase in vitamin C concentrations in these trials (Pitt and Costrin, 1979; Miller *et al.*, 1977). If some therapeutic effect, albeit small, can be realised in these groups where intakes and reserves are considerably above our earlier definition of minimal requirements (intake, 60 mg/day; serum levels, 0.35 mg/100 ml; leucocyte vitamin C, 18 μg/10^8 cells), then what would be the protective effect of vitamin C in those who have relatively poor reserves? This again emphasises the need to maintain intakes and reserves at least above the levels of hypovita-minosis C.

The failure of 1—4 g/day to have any marked effect on the symptoms of the common cold has led to the suggestion that intakes of greater than 10 g/day are required during a viral infection. There are, as yet, no adequately controlled trials assessing the effect of such large intakes, although Anderson (1977) has evidence that intakes of up to 4 g/day during a cold infection are no better than those of 1.5 g at reducing the severity of the symptoms and in addition that there were no significant

differences in the prophylactic effect of doses of 250 mg through to
2 g/day. Because intakes of this order, if taken for long periods, may
have deleterious effects on the body (Chapter 6), we would not
recommend that the healthy ingest 1 g/day or more for periods longer
than one week. We see no reason why those who feel inclined should
not take doses of the order of 1 g at the onset of a cold, as there would
appear to be scientific evidence that such intakes can bring about some
decrease in the severity of the cold symptoms. We see no evidence for
any advantage of continuous therapy of this order and would certainly
not recommend that intakes of greater than 2 g/day be taken either
before or during an infection until there has been more time for the
effects of such intakes, both on the common cold and on the general
metabolism of the body, to be adequately evaluated.

Apart from the common cold, other diseases associated with
persistent infection, and which appear to be primarily a deficiency of
the immune-response mechanisms, have responded well to doses of
vitamin C of the order of 1 g (Anderson and Dittrich, 1979; Boxer
et al., 1979; Rebora, Dallegri and Patrone, 1980), although the
response may not be the same in all individuals and may show some age
dependence (Gallin *et al.*, 1979). The role that vitamin C may play in
such conditions has been considered earlier (Section 3.2.6). In such
diseases, where there is a defect in the immune response, vitamin C may
be found to have a more valuable role than simply the slight beneficial
effect found in protecting the healthy from the worst effects of the
common cold virus. Anderson (1981) has recently reported children
with chronic granulomatous disease to be free of serious infection for
up to three years on 1–2 g of the vitamin per day, an effect which he
attributes to the simple pharmacological reducing properties of the
drug preventing excessive auto-oxidation of the white cells.

5.2 Cardiovascular Disease

The aetiology of cardiovascular disease indicates that a multiplicity of
factors are involved. Although elevated serum lipids are a risk factor,
a causal relationship has not been proven. However, it is thought that
hypercholesterolaemia causes atheromatous change in blood vessels. An
exhaustive review of the experimental evidence for the involvement of
vitamin C in lipid metabolism is beyond the scope of this chapter, but
a suggested role in cholesterol breakdown has been outlined in Section
3.2.1. It would appear that the vitamin is required to maintain adequate

function of the liver's P450-dependent mixed-function oxygenase, which is responsible for the hydroxylation of cholesterol, although the vitamin is not involved directly in the hydroxylation reaction. It has been shown in guinea pigs that latent or chronic vitamin C deficiency (hypovitaminosis C) leads to a decreased activity of this enzyme producing impaired formation of bile acids from cholesterol (Figure 5.1), which results in an increase in tissue and circulating cholesterol

Figure 5.1: Association between Hepatic Vitamin C Concentrations and the Rate of Cholesterol Transformation to Bile Acids in Normal Guinea Pigs (●) and Guinea Pigs with Latent Vitamin C Deficiency (o)

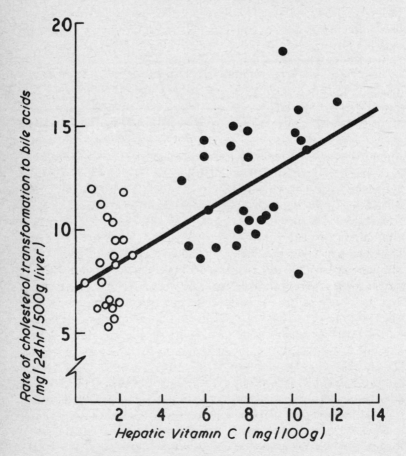

Source: From Ginter (1972).

levels. The important point is that this occurs in chronic vitamin C deficiency and not acute scurvy. Acute scurvy is a complex state, and hence some of the metabolic effects which are observed in vitamin C depleted animals may be due to depletion of other vitamins, to weight loss, anorexia or haemorrhage in addition to low vitamin C reserves (Ginter, 1978). These changes may account for the findings of unaltered or decreased plasma cholesterol levels seen in marked C depletion and scurvy in the human (Bronte-Stewart, Roberts and Wells, 1963; Hodges *et al.*, 1971; Davies and Newson, 1974). Ginter believes that this is an extreme acute effect of gross C depletion on cholesterol synthesis and that it results in a decrease in the body's ability to make cholesterol, with little change in the rate of breakdown of the lipid. Alternatively, decreased excretion or breakdown of cholesterol occurs after several months of hypovitaminosis C when liver enzyme activity falls, but body synthesis of cholesterol remains unaltered (Ginter, 1975).

Ginter and his colleagues (1969) have used a model for hypovitaminosis C which prevents the decreased food consumption and growth seen in scurvy in the guinea pig. The animals are fed a vitamin C deficient diet for two weeks to deplete tissue stores. They are subsequently maintained on 0.5 mg vitamin C daily for as long as 140 days without developing symptoms of scurvy. In such a model, vitamin C depletion has been shown to be accompanied by a rise in serum and liver cholesterol and a deviation of the fatty acid composition of liver cholesterolesters towards an increased proportion of saturated fatty acids (Ginter *et al.*, 1969). It is thought that latent vitamin C deficiency may cause similar biochemical and pathological changes in the human. This claim is based on the findings of Ginter, Kajaba and Nizner (1970), who administered 300 mg vitamin C orally per day to patients with varying levels of serum cholesterol. These workers found that after 47 days there was a statistically significant reduction of serum cholesterol, which was of greatest degree in those who had elevated levels at the start of the trial. Although there are conflicting publications on the effect of C supplementation on the plasma cholesterol levels of man (Turley, West and Horton, 1976; Ginter, 1978), these discrepancies are explained by Ginter (1979b) by the view that C therapy is only effective when cholesterol levels are greater than 200 mg/100 ml and the greater the plasma cholesterol concentration the more effective the C therapy. This suggestion is also supported by earlier reports in the Russian literature (Simonson and Keys, 1961). Evidence that hypovitaminosis C may have significant effects on cholesterol levels in the general population is provided by the seasonal change in plasma cholesterol reflecting inversely the vitamin C levels (Kajaba, 1968).

The evidence that C supplementation is capable of having some effect in the hypercholesterolaemic subject is now gaining acceptance (Geriatrics, Editorial, 1978). Vitamin C may be even more effective than some drugs currently used to treat hypercholesterolaemia (Odumosu and Wilson, 1979). It has also been suggested that vitamin C may be able to mobilise cholesterol from the arterial walls (Spittle, 1973). The findings that high-density lipoproteins, substances believed to aid mobilisation of cholesterol from tissues, are correlated with plasma vitamin C suggests a mechanism for such a function (Bates, Mandal and Cole, 1977). This role, however, remains unproven.

Not only is vitamin C implicated as a hypocholesterolaemic agent, but over the past few years evidence has accumulated suggesting that vitamin C has an effect on the metabolism of triglyceride. Thus, in hyperlipidaemic patients, vitamin C supplements of 2–3 g daily for at least a year appear to be effective in reducing serum triglyceride (Sokoloff *et al.*, 1966). Vitamin C administration (1 g/day) for six months to hyperlipidaemic subjects at the time of seasonal vitamin C deficit brings about a decline in the serum triglyceride of as much as 50 per cent (Ginter, 1976). Massive decreases in circulating triglyceride following vitamin C therapy have also been reported in two patients who had gross hypertriglyceridemias (Geoly and Diamond, 1980). Furthermore, experimental studies have shown that vitamin C deficiency results in hypertriglyceridemia, and this effect may be caused by a decrease in tissue lipolytic activity (Fujinami *et al.*, 1971; Ginter, 1978; Sokoloff *et al.*, 1967; Kotzé and Spies, 1976).

Hyperlipidaemia is not the only factor associated with arterial disease. Degenerative changes in the vessel wall and enhanced clotting tendencies have also been implicated. It is possible that an anti-atherosclerotic activity of vitamin C may also be mediated through these mechanisms as well as by a reduction in blood lipid levels. Vitamin C deficiency could interfere with the metabolism of two important components of the blood vessel wall, collagen and mucopolysaccharides (Section 3.1.1). Changes in collagen and mucopolysaccharide turnover observed in vitamin C deficient arteries (Nambisan and Kurup, 1975; Schwartz and Adamy, 1976) may have a profound effect on the normal structural and permeability characteristics of the arterial wall. Chronic C depletion in animals, without supplementary cholesterol intakes, leads to changes in the vessel wall that resemble atherosclerosis (Willis, 1953, 1957; Sulkin and Sulkin, 1975). The vitamin may also be effective in reducing the incidence of thrombotic episodes. Spittle (1973) divided 60 surgical patients with leg thrombosis into two groups; half received 1 g of vitamin C each day and the rest received a placebo. Using a sensitive radioactive detection method for assessing thrombosis, Spittle found that the incidence of thrombi in the vitamin C supplemented group was only half that in the placebo group. Furthermore, the severity of the thrombi in the supplemented group was much less than in the control patients. Some of this effect may be mediated by increased fibrinolytic activity (Bordia *et al.*, 1978; Bordia, 1980), although it has been suggested that these effects are not long lasting (Crawford *et al.*, 1975). Vitamin C has also been shown to be effective in preventing the fall in fibrinolytic activity which occurs following a fatty meal. The activity, however, remains high only as long as elevated vitamin C levels are maintained, implying adequate administration of the vitamin in divided doses is essential in order to maintain an optimum blood level.

There is circumstantial and indirect evidence that hypovitaminosis C may be a risk factor in arterial disease. There are several studies revealing a close inverse relationship between vitamin C intake and mortality rate in humans (Ginter, 1975; Hanck and Weiser, 1977). A negative correlation between vitamin C intake and standard mortality ratios for cerebrovascular disease and ischaemic heart disease in different regions of the United Kingdom has also been found (Ginter, 1975; Knox, 1973). Deep vein thrombosis and the incidence of ischaemic heart disease are also increased in cold weather, with a spring peak in admission to hospital in the latter group (Dunnigan and Harland, 1970; Lawrence *et al.*, 1977). Such seasonal change shows a remarkable association with the seasonal decrease in blood vitamin C levels (Section 4.1.1). In a recent study (Ramirez and Flowers, 1980), the leucocyte vitamin C levels in patients with coronary arterial disease were found to be significantly lower than those patients without the disease. ECG changes indicative of heart disease are also more frequent in those with poor vitamin C reserves (Cheraskin and Ringsdorf, 1979). In general terms, Clemetson (1979) has noted that many factors which are associated with ischaemic heart disease and thrombosis, such as smoking, infection, soft water and the winter season are also associated with a decrease in circulating vitamin C (Chapter 4). Ginter (1979c) has used this argument to implicate the recent fall in mortality from ischaemic heart disease in the USA with a possible increase in vitamin C reserves encouraged by a decrease in smoking and better dietary practice.

The accumulated evidence suggests that latent vitamin C deficiency (hypovitaminosis C) may be implicated as an aetiological factor in the pathogenesis of coronary artery disease. The possible mechanisms by which vitamin C deficiency exerts its atherogenic effect, involving the liver, blood vessels and tissue is outlined in Figure 5.2. Only long-term, large-scale placebo trials can confirm or refute a role for vitamin C in the prevention of arterial disease, and there would now appear to be sufficient evidence to justify the instigation of such trials, especially as one of the drugs most frequently used for lowering blood lipid levels has recently been found to be more toxic than was originally thought (Oliver *et al.*, 1980).

Figure 5.2: Possible Involvement of Vitamin C Deficiency in the Aetiology of Atherosclerosis

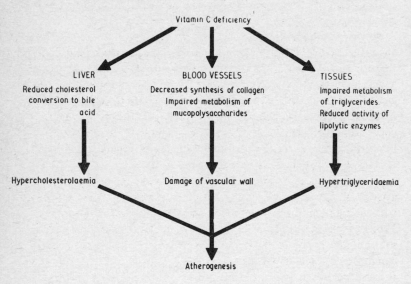

Source: From Ginter *et al.* (1979).

5.3 Malignant Diseases

The aetiology and pathogenesis of cancer is obscure, its treatment is often empirical, and total prevention is not yet feasible. It has long been known that man's food may be involved in the aetiology of certain kinds of cancer. Moreover the natural history of a tumour may be modified by the nutritional status of the host or, conversely, a tumour by reason of its parasitic nature may derange the metabolism of the host because of its own requirements for nutrients. These relationships have been a subject of interest in recent years. This section considers the various relationships of a variety of malignant diseases to a single nutrient, vitamin C. The early work on the use of vitamin C in cancer has been reviewed by Stone (1972) and by Cameron, Pauling and Leibovitz (1979). From these studies it is evident that vitamin C in large doses may have a role in suppressing tumour genesis.

5.3.1 Experimental Evidence

The antitumour activity of vitamin C and its oxidation products has been reported by a number of workers. Ascorbic acid, dehydroascorbic acid and 2,3-diketogulonic acid cause inhibition of growth of the transplanted solid sarcoma-180 in mice, the highest inhibitory activity being shown by dehydroascorbic acid (Yamafuji *et al.*, 1971; Omura *et al.*, 1974). The inhibitory effect of vitamin C seems to be further enhanced by the addition of copper ions as copper sulphate, suggesting that the active agent might be an oxidation product of ascorbic acid. The synergistic effect of copper and vitamin C in inhibiting tumour growth is further evident in a recent *in vitro* study (Bram *et al.*, 1980) involving malignant melanoma cells which are known to be rich in copper (Ikonopisov, 1972). In this study, vitamin C was found to inhibit the growth of the melanoma cells 20–500 times more than normal cells, suggesting selective toxicity of the vitamin.

Several hypotheses have been advanced to explain the antitumour activity of vitamin C in the presence of copper ions. Copper ions react with vitamin C and generate free radicals in solution (Peloux *et al.*, 1962) which, in turn, leads to reductions in the viscosity of DNA solutions (Yamafuji *et al.*, 1971). It is possible, therefore, that the carcinostatic effect of vitamin C is mediated by interaction with DNA. It has also been suggested that dehydroascorbic acid functions as an electron acceptor in the regulation of mitosis (Edgar, 1970).

Benade, Howard and Burk (1969) observed a synergistic killing of Ehrlich ascites carcinoma cells *in vitro* by vitamin C and 3-amino-1,2,4-triazole. Their experimental results indicated that vitamin C is lethal to Ehrlich ascites carcinoma cells and harmless to normal cells. The effect of vitamin C is probably influenced by intracellular generation of toxic H_2O_2 produced by oxidation of the vitamin (Equation 3.5), which is more deleterious to tumour cells because of their low catalase activity compared with normal tissues (Orr, 1970).

High-dose vitamin C in mice is reported to reduce colo-rectal tumour development from rectal polyps in susceptible inbred strains (Logue and Frommer, 1980) and also to reduce the number of potentially pre-malignant polyps in the human with familial polyposis (De Cosse *et al.*, 1975). Schlegel *et al.* (1969, 1970) have shown that vitamin C can prevent the formation of spontaneous bladder tumours in mice. They studied 3-hydroxyanthranilic acid (3-HOA), a metabolite of tryptophan, as a possible urinary carcinogen. Oral administration of large amounts of vitamin C (added to the drinking water) prevented the carcinogenic effect of 3-HOA pellets implanted into mice bladders. It was thought that vitamin C affinity for oxygen prevented the oxidation of 3-HOA, since it is the oxidation product rather than the compound itself that is carcinogenic. However, several studies contradicted this suggested role of 3-HOA in tumourgenesis, especially in humans. Thus, Benassi, Perissiotto and Allegri (1963) found low urinary concentrations of 3-HOA in the urine of bladder tumour patients. In another study, Price *et al.* (1960) observed that only about 50 per cent of their patients with bladder cancer excreted urine with high concentrations of the tryptophan metabolite. Nevertheless, according to Schlegel (1975), the spontaneous oxidation of 3-HOA and subsequently the incidence of bladder cancer can be reduced by daily oral intake of 1.5 g of vitamin C.

Histochemical examination has shown that vitamin C is mobilised and made available for organs and tissues which show a high rate of metabolism or cell division (Tomutti, 1937, 1938). This might be the reason for the increased levels of vitamin C in tumour tissue compared to normal surrounding tissue (Moriarty *et al.*, 1977). It has been established that vitamin C synthesis in rats and mice can be evoked by exposure to various compounds including the carcinogenic hydrocarbons (Boyland and Grover, 1961; Conney and Burns, 1959). If vitamin C is utilised by tumour tissues, the amount of the vitamin available to the surrounding normal tissue may be reduced which, in turn, may reduce the effectiveness of the host's resistance.

It appears that most of the experimental studies of the effect of vitamin C on the incidence, induction and growth of tumours have been carried out in species, such as rats and mice, which possess the ability to synthesise vitamin C. For direct comparison with man, however, the guinea pig or other primates should be the experimental animal of choice. Unfortunately, such tumour model systems are not in common use, and the available evidence is both fragmentary and contradictory. Migliozzi (1977) used methylcholanthrene-induced guinea pig sarcoma as his experimental model. Complete tumour regression occurred in 55 per cent of those animals receiving 0.3 mg/kg/day vitamin C, whereas animals given 10 mg/kg/day showed tumour inhibition but no regression. In contrast, tumours in animals maintained on 1 g/kg/day grew without sign of retardation. Furthermore, all tumour-bearing animals previously maintained on 1 g/kg/day vitamin C died within 21 days when given 0.3 mg/kg. It seems, therefore, that much more research is needed in order to investigate the antitumour activity of vitamin C, especially using animals which, like humans, are incapable of synthesising the vitamin.

Not only is there experimental evidence for a direct effect of vitamin C on the malignant cell, but research has also suggested that the vitamin may reduce the carcinogenic potential of some chemicals. In recent years there appears to be substantial evidence suggesting that a variety of experimental tumours of the alimentary tract, liver, lung and bladder can be produced by nitroso compounds (Mirvish, 1971; Mirvish *et al.*, 1975; Narisawa *et al.*, 1976; Rustia, 1975), which are produced by the reaction of nitrites with secondary and tertiary amines, amides or ureas:

$$(R_1, R_2)-N-H + HNO_2 \rightleftharpoons (R_1, R_2)-N - N = O + H_2O \quad \text{(Eq. 5.1)}$$

In 1972, Mirvish and his associates reported that the nitrosation of several secondary and tertiary amines can be blocked *in vitro* by the addition of vitamin C. The amines studied were oxytetracycline, morpholine, piperazine, *N*-methylamine and dimethylamine. More recently, experiments with rats have shown that the vitamin also exerts a protective effect against hepatotoxicity following oral administration of sodium nitrite and aminopyrine (Kamm *et al.*, 1973). Hepatotoxicity in this case is believed to be due to formation of dimethylnitrosamine by the reaction of nitrous acid with aminopyrine.

It has been suggested that the potential hazard of ingesting drugs or food containing nitrites and secondary amines which can be nitrosated may be prevented by the addition of vitamin C (Mirvish *et al.*, 1972). Indeed, Fiddler and his co-workers (1973) have demonstrated that addition of the vitamin to the ingredients used to cure frankfurters greatly reduces the formation of dimethylnitrosamine. Raineri and Weisburger (1975) demonstrated that under simulated gastric conditions (37°, pH 1.5), a vitamin C/nitrite molar ratio of 4:1 provided 93 per cent protection from *in vitro* nitrosation of methylurea (Table 5.1).

What is the mechanism for this vitamin C effect? When incubated under simulated gastric conditions, vitamin C appears to react directly

Table 5.1: Effect of Vitamin C on the Formation of Methylnitrosourea in Potato Incubated with Nitrite and Methylurea under Simulated Gastric Conditions (37°, pH 1.5). Five gram samples of homogenised boiled potato were used.

Vitamin C/Nitrite (Molar Ratio)	Nitrite (% Decrease)	Methylnitrosourea (% Inhibition)
0/1	0	0
1/1	13	37
2/1	36	74
4/1	43	93

Source: Modified data from Raineri and Weisburger (1975).

with the nitrite in potato yielding a 43 per cent decrease in nitrite concentration and there was no evidence that the vitamin reacted with methylurea or the product methylnitrosourea (Raineri and Weisburger, 1975). Vitamin C does not seem to react with amines, nor does it increase the rate of nitrosamine decomposition; it reacts very rapidly with nitrite and nitrous acid, however (Archer *et al.*, 1975). It is possible that the vitamin lowers the amount of available nitrite by reducing nitrous acid to nitrogen oxides (Equation 5.2) and consequently inhibiting the N-nitrosation reaction (Equation 5.1).

$$2HNO_2 + \text{ascorbate} \longrightarrow \text{dehydroascorbate} + 2NO + 2H_2O$$

(Eq. 5.2)

Further evidence for the protective effect of vitamin C in carcinogenesis induced by nitrosamine formation was provided by Guttemplan (1977). Using the Ames test, this worker demonstrated that vitamin C inhibits bacterial mutagenesis by N-methyl-N-nitroguanidine, mutagenesis being a change which could potentially lead to carcinogenesis in the animal cell.

In summary, experimental evidence suggests that vitamin C may not only directly inhibit tumour growth, but also modify potential carcinogens to less harmful compounds thus reducing the probability of initiating a malignancy.

5.3.2 Clinical Evidence

As is the case in many chronic diseases (Section 4.2.2), there have been a number of reports suggesting that the majority of patients with malignant disease have minimal tissue stores of vitamin C (Table 5.2)

Table 5.2: Leucocyte Vitamin C Levels in Patients with Malignant Disease

Type of Cancer (Number of Patients)	Mean Leucocyte Vitamin C (μg/10^8 WBC)		Reference
	Control	Cancer	
Miscellaneous cancers (50)	29.5	11.5	Krasner and Dymock (1974)
Miscellaneous cancers (24)	24.3	11.2	Cameron (1975)
Miscellaneous cancers (26)	33.8	17.6	Basu *et al.* (1974)
Advanced breast cancers (22)	33.8	10.8	Basu *et al.* (1974)
Leukaemia (42)	35.0	8.2	Waldo and Zipf (1955)
Acute lymphatic leukaemia (10)	56.4	35.9	Kakar, Wilson and Bell (1975)

and many of these patients have associated physical signs of sub-clinical scurvy (hypovitaminosis C) such as haemorrhage. There is evidence to suggest that the patients with metastatic cancer have increased requirements for the vitamin. Thus an early study revealed that the patients with metastatic cancer utilise twice as much vitamin C as either the control subjects or the patients with localised cancer (Minor and Ramirez, 1943).

During the past few years, several nonrandomised studies have suggested that oral administration of vitamin C in large doses (10 g/day) may be useful in the management of patients with malignant disease. Cameron and Campbell (1974) studied 50 such patients who had not received chemotherapy and reported tumour regression in five of these subjects. In a later report, 50 patients who had previously received irradiation and chemotherapy were combined with the first group, and the survival of all 100 patients was compared with that of 1,000 control cases selected retrospectively from the records at the Vale of Leven Hospital, Scotland (Cameron and Pauling, 1976). For each vitamin C treated patient, ten controls were matched on the basis of age, sex, site and histological features of the primary tumour. The mean survival of patients given vitamin C was 210 days, compared with only 50 for the selected controls. In another report, Cameron and Pauling (1978) provided evidence that the mean survival of patients given vitamin C was greater than 293 days, compared with only 38 for the controls.

In 1978, Morishige and Murata reported results of another nonrandomised trial involving 99 patients with terminal cancer who had been admitted to the Fukuoka Torikai Hospital, Japan. Of the patients, 44 received 4 g or less of vitamin C per day (low vitamin C) and 55 received 5 g or more (high vitamin C). The mean survival of patients given low vitamin C was found to be 43 days, compared with 246 days for the high vitamin C supplemented patients. Six of the high vitamin C patients were still alive when the report was written, with an average survival of 866 days. The results of this nonrandomised clinical trial appear to be in agreement with those of Cameron and Pauling (1976, 1978) and indicate that supplemental vitamin C in large doses has significant beneficial effects on patients with advanced cancer. Not only is life expectancy increased in patients in these studies, but improvement in their state of well-being has also been indicated by better appetite, increased mental alertness and desire to return to normal life.

The findings of these nonrandomised trials gained further support from an *in vitro* study reported by Bishun and his colleagues (1978). In this study, biopsy materials from an epidermoid carcinoma of the mouth of a 54-year-old caucasion were grown in culture, and subsequently a stable line of epidermoid carcinomatous cells was established. Using this stable line of the carcinomatous cells in culture, it was demonstrated that the addition of vitamin C (600 μg/ml or more) resulted in an increased ratio of dead to live cells and a decreased rate of DNA synthesis.

The value of supplemental vitamin C in cancer management has been reassessed in a recent study (Creagan *et al.*, 1979) through a properly designed placebo-clinical trial involving 123 advanced cancer patients. The patients were divided randomly into a group that received 10 g of vitamin C per day and one that received a lactose placebo. This controlled double-blind study, however, failed to show any appreciable difference in survival time and general well-being between the two groups of patients.

Although available evidence indicates that supplemental vitamin C could produce substantial benefits in both the prevention and the treatment of cancer, the subject still remains controversial, especially after the negative findings of Creagan's placebo-controlled trial. The role of vitamin C in cancer must be refuted or supported by adequately controlled studies using multi-centre programmes which would eliminate any bias in the outcome of the results. Such studies of vitamin C and cancer become of even greater significance when it is appreciated that much of the current chemotherapy has been shown to be unsuccessful in prolonging survival time of cancer patients (Powels *et al.*, 1980).

5.4 Skeletal Disorders

In recent years there have been reports claiming that large doses of vitamin C produce relief of skeletal pain in various disorders. These conditions are bone metastases, Paget's disease of bone and osteogenesis imperfecta.

5.4.1 Skeletal Metastases

In the course of a clinical trial, Cameron and Baird (1973) observed pain relief in a group of patients with multiple skeletal metastases, when administered 10 g of vitamin C daily for about one week. These workers also claimed that regular narcotic analgesic treatment could be discontinued in these patients without inducing withdrawal symptoms. It has been shown that urinary hydroxyproline (UHP) levels in patients with breast cancer are directly proportional to the degree of ossious deposits (Cuschieri, 1973; Basu, Donaldson and Williams, 1974). The skeletal metastases are known to cause bone resorption, and this involves extensive loss of bone matrix. It is, therefore, possible that the increased level of UHP in the patients with breast tumour and skeletal metastases may be due to an increased rate of degradation of bone collagen rather than a direct effect of the primary breast tumour itself. However, in a study carried out by Basu and his co-workers (1974) it was evident that the UHP levels in breast cancer patients with skeletal metastases bear an inverse relationship to leucocyte vitamin C levels (Table 5.3) and that a loading dose of 1 g of vitamin C produces a sharp decrease in UHP excretion.

Thus, it appears that invasive neoplastic cells possess the ability to disrupt pre-existing collagen barriers, with increased collagen catabolism resulting in an increased output of hydroxyproline residues, and this disruptive effect can be diminished by increasing vitamin C intake. These results may prove to have practical implications for the treatment of patients with bone metastases. However, large-scale clinical trials along such lines have yet to be undertaken.

5.4.2 Paget's Disease of Bone

Paget's disease of bone is characterised by excessive osteoclastic and osteoblastic activity leading to pain and bone deformity. The treatment of this disease has been centred upon the use of analgesics and drugs which suppress the increased resorption and formation of bone. Of the latter, the major agent in clinical use is calcitonin, and treatment with this compound is well documented (Kanis *et al.*, 1974). Calcitonin is

Table 5.3: Leucocyte Vitamin C and Urinary Hydroxyproline Levels

Group (Number of Subjects)	Leucocyte Ascorbic Acid ($\mu g/10^8$ WBC)	Urinary Hydroxyproline (mg/g creatinine)
Healthy subjects (10)	33.8	15.8
Miscellaneous cancers (26) (without skeletal deposits)	17.6	46.6
Breast cancer (22) (with skeletal deposits)	10.8	138.0

known to inhibit osteoclastic activity, resulting in a reduced UHP excretion and there is also relief of pain, but the patients vary considerably in their response. Furthermore, calcitonin is very expensive.

In a clinical trial in which sixteen patients with Paget's disease of bone were given one gram of vitamin C three times daily, eight patients experienced a decrease of pain within five to seven days after commencing the treatment (Basu *et al.*, 1978). In three of these patients, pain was completely abolished. Of the remaining thirteen patients who were subsequently treated with calcitonin, four had total and seven had partial relief of pain, whilst two, in whom the pain was not entirely due to Paget's disease but rather to secondary arthritis, experienced no relief.

It must be emphasised that this was a short-term trial. The long-term effects of treatment with vitamin C await clinical, radiological and biochemical review. From the patient's point of view, the relief of pain is an important factor for it is this that causes him to visit his doctor. If pain can be alleviated or even abolished by cheap, easily produced drugs which can be taken orally, like vitamin C, this is to be preferred to embarking immediately on an expensive course of injections with calcitonin. However, the use of vitamin C should not prevent subsequent therapy with calcitonin if this leads to the greater radiological and biochemical improvement of Paget's disease.

5.4.3 Osteogenesis Imperfecta

Osteogenesis imperfecta is a metabolic bone disorder characterised by fractures following minor trauma, often associated with development of bony deformities. In a clinical study involving ten patients (aged 5–27 years), vitamin C was chosen as a possible therapeutic agent, the dose being 1 g daily (Winterfeldt, Eyring and Vivian, 1970). This study revealed that all treated patients experienced a decreased number of fractures when compared with the untreated. It was also noted that a decrease in UHP excretion was observed after a period of three months in six of the ten patients, indicating either an increased deposition of more stable collagen or a decreased collagen degradation. The beneficial effect of vitamin C on osteogenesis imperfecta was further evident in another clinical study (Kurz and Eyring, 1974) involving 13 patients aged from birth to 15 years. This study demonstrated not only a significant decrease in fractures, but also a marked improvement in physical activity.

5.5 Tissue Healing

It is well recognised that wound healing requires synthesis and accumulation of collagen and subsequent cross-linking of the fibres to give new tensile strength to the damaged tissue. Of significance in this context is the fact that vitamin C has a critical role in wound repair and especially in participating as a co-factor in the hydroxylation of specific peptidyl-proline and peptidyl-lysine residues during collagen biosynthesis (Section 3.1.1).

There appears to be substantial experimental evidence suggesting that adequate supplies of vitamin C are necessary for the normal healing process. Thus, an early study (Bourne, 1946) demonstrated that maximum tensile strength of scar tissue in guinea pigs was achieved when vitamin C was fed at 2 mg/kg/day, three to four times the level necessary to prevent scurvy. However, when very high doses of the vitamin (30 mg/day) were used, no added beneficial effect was observed. A similar observation was made in a more recent study, where Yew (1973) showed that guinea pigs receiving 0.5 mg/kg/day exhibited very slow wound healing in comparison with those receiving 5 mg/kg/day, and that increasing the dose of the vitamin from 5 to 500 mg did not encourage more rapid healing.

Reports of low blood vitamin C levels in postoperative patients (Bartlett, Jones and Ryan, 1940; Crandon *et al.*, 1961; Shukla, 1969) have led to the suggestion that deficiency of the vitamin may be an important factor in the pathogenesis of postoperative wound complications in surgical patients (Crandon *et al.*, 1961). It has been suggested that there is rapid utilisation of vitamin C for the synthesis of collagen at the site of the wound in the postoperative period, and hence the administration of the vitamin postoperatively might be beneficial (Shukla, 1969). Using 150 surgical patients, Coon (1962) was able to show that at least 200 mg vitamin C/day would be required to maintain

postoperative blood concentrations of vitamin C at an adequate level
(0.4 mg/100 ml).

Vitamin C has also been reported to promote healing of pressure
sores. Thus, Hunter and Rajan (1971) found a deficiency of the vitamin
in paraplegic and tetraplegic patients with sores. Tissue biopsies of the
edge of the sores showed an increased collagen content in patients
supplemented with vitamin C. In patients recovering from surgery who
had sustained bed sores, Taylor and his associates (1974), through a
double-blind trial, demonstrated a faster reduction in pressure sore
area when 1 g/day of vitamin C was given for one month.

There is evidence that vitamin C may also promote healing of burns.
Thus, Klasson (1951) found that large doses of vitamin C could
alleviate pain, shorten the healing period and reduce the time interval
necessary for grafting in five male subjects with severe burns. He
advocates the use of 1 g of vitamin C to be administered intravenously
in an electrolyte solution during the first hours after burns occur. In a
more recent report, Klenner (1971) advocates the use of much higher
doses of vitamin C in patients with burns to accelerate healing and
alleviate pain. However, in experimental studies in man (Section 4.3.1),
considerable depletion of tissue vitamin C is required before wounds
fail to heal properly. In summary therefore, it must be said that, with
the possible exception of certain types of wound such as the bed sore,
research in both animals and humans indicates that large doses of
vitamin C do not encourage more rapid tissue healing than the smaller
intakes required to prevent hypovitaminosis C (60 mg/day).

5.6 Hypersensitivity

Early studies have indicated that large doses of vitamin C may be
effective against allergic reactions to a number of substances, including
ragweed pollen (Holmes and Alexander, 1942; Pelner, 1944), sulpho-
namides (Holmes, 1943; Schropp, 1943) and arsphenamines (Cormia,
1941; Delp, 1941). There is also evidence that patients exhibiting
hypersensitivity to some of these substances have associated low blood
vitamin C levels (Friend and Marquis, 1938; Vail, 1941). It has been
suggested that the low blood levels are the result of the toxic reaction
rather than a predisposing factor to such reactions. Holmes (1943) has
observed that the rate of urinary vitamin C excretion in a group of
healthy subjects increases to 2–3 times the normal level following
administration of 30 grains of sulphathiazole.

In a more recent study (Anah, Jarike and Baig, 1980), a double-blind trial was carried out in which administration of vitamin C, the dose being 1 g/day for 14 weeks, was found to be effective against asthma in reducing severity and frequency of asthmatic attacks. It was also shown that this effect was reversed when vitamin C therapy ceased. The therapeutic effect of vitamin C in asthma was further supported by observations made in guinea pigs showing that the vitamin protects these animals against anaphylactic shock (Dawson and West, 1965).

The ventilatory function is measured by recording partial expiratory flow-volume (PEFV) curves in order to assess the degree of airway constriction induced by pharmacological agents (Bouhuys *et al.*, 1969). In general, decreased flow rates reflect airway constriction, while increased flows indicate dilatation of small airpassages. Using this technique, it has been shown that a single oral dose of 500 mg vitamin C inhibits the constrictor effect of histamine on the airpassage of human subjects, and that this effect lasts for at least six hours (Zuskin, Lewis and Bouhuys, 1973). Experiments with anaesthetised guinea pigs have also revealed that vitamin C has a direct relaxant effect on airway smooth muscle (Zuskin, Lewis and Bouhuys, 1973).

Indeed, there is evidence (Busieno, 1949; Dawson and West, 1965) to suggest that not only does vitamin C antagonise histamine but also histamine depresses the vitamin content of the adrenal cortex. It appears that vitamin C in large doses may be beneficial to patients with certain types of allergic reactions, and that this effect may be mediated through lowering body histamine levels. However, the mechanism by which vitamin C interacts with histamine is not yet understood, and awaits further studies.

5.7 Periodontal Disease

It is a physiological fact that the periodontium is in a continual state of flux. Thus, the bone and cementum are constantly remodelling to accommodate the stress of mastication and occlusion, and these complementary depositions and resorptions of cementum maintain the constant thickness of the periodontal membrane. Autoradiographic studies with tritiated proline show a constant renewal of collagen in the periodontium, which relies on vitamin C (Carneiro and Fava de Moraes, 1965).

An investigation of vitamin C deficient guinea pigs has shown that the periodontal membrane is associated with structural disruption, the severest changes being in the area adjacent to alveolar bone (Glickman, 1948a). This area appears to be completely devoid of well-formed collagenous fibres, and the space is filled with haemorrhage and detached remnants of degenerated collagen. Glickman (1948b) also described the effect of artificially induced inflammation on vitamin C deficient guinea pigs. He applied 10 per cent silver nitrate to the labile gingiva for 30 seconds in deficient and control animals. In the deficient animals, the non-irritated tissue showed the same breakdown of periodontal membrane and indentation seen in the scorbutic state, but the irritated tissue showed even more severe collagen breakdown in the membrane. On the other hand, in the control animals the collagen degeneration was only slight in the irritated area. These findings support the argument that while vitamin C deficiency does not cause gingival inflammation, the local irritating factor which does produce it will cause increased destruction when there is vitamin C deficiency.

In a more recent study (Cowan, 1976), a double-blind trial was carried out investigating the high-dose (1 g/day) effect of vitamin C on the periodontal membrane space in a group of young patients. This study showed an improvement of the areas of irregularity in the membrane shadow of a significant number of vitamin C treated cases as compared with controls.

5.8 Vitamin-sparing Effect

Vitamin C has been found to have protective power against deficiencies of a number of vitamins, including thiamin, riboflavin, pantothenic acid, biotin, folic acid (Section 3.1.2), cyanocobalamine, retinol and α-tocopherol (Terroine, 1960). The demonstration of this protective power has been primarily based on experimental observations, which include growth rate, survival time, appetite, clinical symptoms and metabolic signs in animals fed a vitamin-deficient diet with or without vitamin C supplements.

Recently, some workers have attempted to highlight the mechanism of the protective power of vitamin C against thiamin deficiency (Murdock, Donaldson and Gubler, 1974). These workers showed that thiamin-deficient rats with an oral supplement of vitamin C (5 per cent) had nearly normal growth rate, and those injected sub-cutaneously with vitamin C grew only slightly better than the thiamin-deficient rats with no supplement. Thus, these results indicate that sub-cutaneous administration with vitamin C has no thiamin-sparing effect but that there is an effect when vitamin C is given orally. These workers also demonstrated that the thiamin-deficient rats with an oral supplement of vitamin C had nearly normal levels of thiamin in the faeces. On the basis of these results, it has been claimed that the thiamin-sparing effect of vitamin C may be due to stimulation of biosynthesis of thiamin by the gut microflora which then may become available to the rats, largely via coprophagy.

More recently, the thiamin-sparing effect of vitamin C has been demonstrated in humans (Basu, Jenner and Williams, 1976). This study was carried out in 16 female geriatric patients who were deficient in thiamin as determined by measuring the thiamin pyrophosphate stimulating effect (TPP effect) on transketolase enzyme activity in their haemolysed red blood cells. Oral administration of vitamin C (3 g/day) for one week resulted not only in a decreased 'TPP effect' but also in increased urinary excretory levels of thiamin.

These results, however, do not support the hypothesis that thiamin synthesised by the gut microflora becomes available to the rats via coprophagy. One may perhaps speculate that vitamin C decreases the need for thiamin by supplying metabolites by non-thiamin-requiring pathways. This may account for the fact that the urinary excretory level of thiamin was increased by oral supplementation with vitamin C in the human. This speculation, however, does not explain the reduction in the 'TPP effect'. The mechanism of the thiamin-sparing effect of vitamin C still remains far from clear.

5.9 Conclusions

Very high intakes of vitamin C of the order of 500 mg/day are not without hazard (Chapter 6). Such toxic effects, however, are unlikely to manifest themselves unless individuals are on high intakes for considerable periods of time. We therefore see no reason why individuals who so choose should not take 1 or 2 g per day during the first few days of a common cold infection. It is unlikely that in the majority of people this will have a marked effect on symptoms but it may lead to some decrease in the severity of the side effects. High dosage of vitamin C may also be appropriate in some individuals who suffer from chronic infections due to immune deficiency disease and some types of asthma.

Whether high-dose vitamin C therapy is going to be effective in the treatment or prevention of cancer and arterial disease has yet to be ascertained. There would appear to be definite hopes that vitamin C treatment may bring about some reduction in risk in developing arterial disease. However, such evidence will take a considerable time to collect owing to the fact that the degenerative changes seen in arterial disease take many years to develop. In the intervening period whilst suitable evidence is being collected, again we see no reason why those who so wish should not take vitamin C daily at a rate up to 200 mg/day. Such intakes can be obtained from the normal diet by adequate consumption of fruit and fresh vegetables, including potatoes, provided that the latter are adequately prepared (Chapter 4).

We hesitate to recommend large doses (above 200 mg/day) of vitamin C for the whole of the population because, as yet, we feel that although there are indications, there is no confirmatory evidence that they are beneficial. All the evidence in this chapter, however, adds weight to the conclusions of the previous section that, at the very least, intakes in the order of 60 mg/day should be maintained in normal healthy individuals.

6 SAFETY CONSIDERATIONS ON HIGH INTAKE OF VITAMIN C

In recent years, vitamin C in large doses (1–20 g per day) has been claimed to have prophylactic and therapeutic effects in many patholo-gical conditions (Chapter 5). As a consequence of these claims, the vitamin is taken by many individuals in large doses, 1–5 g per day as opposed to the usual dietary requirement of 30–60 mg. The use of massive doses of vitamin C has not been criticised in the same way as has the use of excessive doses of fat-soluble vitamins, since the body has the capacity to excrete rapidly the water-soluble vitamin (Figure 2.4). Indeed there are a number of isolated reports (Abt and Farmer, 1938; Lowry, Bessey and Burch, 1952; Stone, 1967; Herjanic and Moss-Herjanic, 1967; Klenner, 1971) claiming that vitamin C taken in megadoses has no adverse effects. However, concern has been expressed with regard to the potential hazard of prolonged and regular ingestion of large amounts of the vitamin..This chapter outlines the evidence supporting the fact that vitamin C in large doses may not be as innocuous as is generally believed.

6.1 Growth and Mortality Rate

Megadoses of vitamin C have been reported to result in retardation of growth in experimental animals. Thus, Nandi and his associates (1973) demonstrated that the daily administration of 50 mg vitamin C to guinea pigs fed a wheat flour diet resulted in a significant decrease in growth, compared to that obtained on 5–20 mg of the vitamin per day, and was accompanied by 50 per cent mortality in 16 days and 100 per cent mortality in 25 days. With 100 mg of vitamin C, the effect was more drastic and all animals died within 16 days. Supplementation of this wheat diet by lysine, an essential amino acid found only in low concentrations in wheat, counteracted the toxicity of the large doses of the vitamin.

It is of further interest that the administration of vitamin C (3 g/day for three successive days) to five healthy volunteers, has been shown to reduce the urinary excretion of lysine to less than 50 per cent of pre-vitamin C values (Basu, 1979). Thus it may be that the findings with

115

guinea pigs (Nandi *et al.*, 1973) are applicable to human beings, so that in countries where the diet consists mainly of cereals, intake of large doses of vitamin C may be harmful. Other workers (Sorensen, Devine and Rivers, 1974; Yew, 1973) also found that guinea pigs treated with megadoses of vitamin C had a reduced growth rate compared to animals fed a normal diet. There are, however, many studies which reveal no such effects (Lamden and Schweiker, 1955; Hornig *et al.*, 1973).

6.2 Protein and Amino Acid Metabolism

Vitamin C is, in part, metabolised to vitamin C-sulphate in man (Section 1.5), the sulphate being derived from sulphur-containing amino acids, such as cysteine. Sulphate formation is also an important pathway in the conjugation and excretion of many drugs (Basu, 1980). This pathway of sulphate conjugation is subject to competitive inhibition when supplies of sulphur are minimal. Houston and Levy (1975) have shown that when vitamin C in large doses is taken with salicylamide there is a decrease in salicylamide sulphate produced and a corresponding increase in glucuronide production. These results indicate that at high dosage vitamin C may compete with certain drugs for sulphate conjugation, which could affect the pharmacological activity and toxicity of drugs.

More recent studies have demonstrated that the oral administration of vitamin C (3 g/day) for three successive days to six healthy volunteers reduces the excretion of cysteine in the urine to 50 per cent of pre-vitamin C values (Basu, 1977), and this may be due to the fact that the amino acid is utilised to metabolise this vitamin. Experimental and clinical evidence (Wokes, 1958; Smith, 1961) suggests that the detoxification of cyanide received from various sources (Wilson and Langman, 1966), takes place by its conversion to a sulphur-containing metabolite, thiocyanate, and that this reaction may require cysteine. It is of interest that the urinary levels of thiocyanate have also been found to be markedly decreased by administration of high doses of vitamin C, whilst the concomitant administration of cysteine (10 mg/ day) restored the urinary thiocyanate to normal levels (Basu, 1977). Thus, when excess vitamin C is ingested and the protein intake is limited, it is possible that cysteine would be monopolised for sulphate conjugation by the vitamin, and as a consequence render one of the body's detoxification mechanisms less effective.

Megadoses of vitamin C have also been reported to affect uric acid metabolism in man. Thus, Stein, Hasan and Fox (1976) found that 4 g daily doses of the vitamin caused a two-fold increase in uric acid excretion and a decrease in blood urate concentration. These workers suggested that the vitamin C induced uricosuria was due to a decrease in the binding of urate to plasma proteins.

Uric acid is the end product of purine base catabolism and purines require amino acids for their formation. Increased uric acid excretion may therefore be another route by which vitamin C leads to depletion of body nitrogen. Furthermore, the excessive renal tubular uric acid may also lead to the precipitation of urate stones, especially as uric acid will be less soluble in the acid urine which will be produced during high vitamin C intake. In addition, vitamin C intake in large amounts could invalidate studies involving the measurement of plasma uric acid and obscure the diagnosis of conditions such as gout. It is, however, necessary to emphasise that many individuals taking megadoses of the vitamin do not appear to manifest uricosuria (unpublished observation).

6.3 Oxalate Excretion

Vitamin C is partly metabolised to oxalic acid which is excreted in the urine (Section 1.5). A number of workers have cautioned that regular ingestion of large amounts of vitamin C may have adverse effects attributable to increased oxalic acid excretion (Lamden and Chrystowski, 1954; Lamden, 1971; Briggs, Gracia-Webb and Davies, 1973). It has been suggested that the greater the quantity of oxalate excreted, the greater the probability of calcium oxalate calculi formation, and therefore that intake of vitamin C in large doses may lead to the formation of renal stones. Nevertheless, the effect of the vitamin on oxalate excretion, like that on urate, is subject to considerable individual variation. This may account for the fact that many workers have failed to note any significant increase in oxalate excretion on administration of up to 5 g daily of vitamin C for up to five years (Atkins *et al.*, 1963; Takiguchi, Furuyama and Shimazono, 1966; Murphy and Zelman, 1965).

6.4 Gastrointestinal Disturbances

There have been several reports (Goldsmith, 1971; Hume, Johnstone and Weyers, 1972; Regnier, 1968) in the literature stating that mega vitamin C intake results in gastrointestinal discomfort characterised by nausea, abdominal cramps, heartburn and diarrhoea. Such disturbances are perhaps the most consistent abnormalities noted in subjects taking the vitamin in gram quantities. The vitamin C associated disturbances, however, may be ameliorated or eliminated by taking the vitamin either with meals or as the sodium salt.

6.5 Lysis of Erythrocytes

The administration of large doses of vitamin C to volunteers has been found to result in increased susceptibility of red cells to haemolysis. The subjects with glucose-6-phosphate dehydrogenase deficiency are especially susceptible to this adverse affect of megadoses of the vitamin (Mengel and Greene, 1976). This is supported by a report of megadose vitamin C therapy contributing to the death of a negro who was deficient in the glucose-6-phosphate dehydrogenase enzyme (Campbell, Steinberg and Bower, 1975). The individual concerned was a 60-year-old man with acute renal failure following second degree burns for which he had been treated intravenously with 80 g of vitamin C per day, for two days. Following treatment with the vitamin, the patient became oliguric with extensive haemolysis and marked urinary excretion of haemoglobin (4 mg/100 ml). The patient died on the twenty-second day following treatment with vitamin C.

6.6 Interaction with Warfarin

There have been a few reports in the literature suggesting that the administration of vitamin C shortens the prothrombin time in animals receiving warfarin anticoagulants (Sigell and Flessa, 1970). A similar effect was noted in a few isolated clinical cases (Rosenthal, 1971; Hume, Johnstone and Weyers, 1972; Smith *et al.*, 1972). This interaction of vitamin C with warfarin appears to be inconsistent (Feetam, Leach and Meynell, 1975). However, it is recognised that vitamin C in large doses can increase the rate of metabolism and excretion of several drugs probably by its effect on the liver cytochome P450-dependent mixed-function oxygenase system (Section 3.2.1). A reduced effectiveness of some drugs due to increased metabolism stimulated by high vitamin C intake may be as important a consideration as the prolonged activity of some drugs occurring during vitamin C deficiency.

6.7 Destruction of Vitamin B_{12}

In 1974, Herbert and Jacob reported that increasing levels of vitamin C added to homogenised meals prior to incubation at $37°C$ for 30 minutes as a laboratory mimic of the gastric environment in man, produced increasing destruction of vitamin B_{12}. However, these workers measured B_{12} in food by a method which was developed for assays of the vitamin in serum, where mild extraction appeared to be adequate. Since vitamin B_{12} in food, unlike serum, is usually tightly bound to proteins, it is essential that methods involving extensive extraction procedures which will release the bound vitamin, are used for assaying B_{12} content of food. Indeed, using one of these methods, Newmark *et al.* (1976) showed that there were no significant deleterious effects of added vitamin C on vitamin B_{12} stability in foods.

It is known, however, that pure hydroxycobalamin and cyanocobalamin are destroyed by vitamin C in the presence of oxygen and copper ions. In a recent study, Herbert *et al.*, (1978) have found low serum B_{12} levels in patients receiving 2 g vitamin C daily for varying periods of time. Subnormal serum B_{12} concentrations have also been shown in healthy subjects who had been taking at least 1 g vitamin C daily for over three years (Hines, 1975). In view of the available evidence, it has been suggested that regular evaluation of B_{12} status is essential in anyone taking more than 0.5 grams of vitamin C daily (Herbert *et al.*, 1978). In contrast Hogenkamp (1980), reviewing the information available, has concluded that it is unlikely that megadose vitamin C intake will destroy a large proportion of the cobalamins in the serum and stores of the healthy, but it may be harmful in those suffering from inborn errors of B_{12} metabolism.

6.8 Bone Metabolism

Vitamin C is known to be required for the synthesis of the major components of the bone matrix, collagen and possibly mucopolysaccharides (Section 3.1.1). On this basis, one would expect large intakes of the vitamin to have little effect on the metabolism of bone. Work from several laboratories shows that this may not be the case, and in fact large doses of vitamin C may have untoward effects. Thus supplementary vitamin C, 220 mg/kg of diet, has been reported to lead to increased mobilisation of calcium and phosphorus from the skeleton of chicks (Thornton, 1970). Brown, Sharma and Young (1971) examined the influence of large doses of vitamin C on excretion of hydroxyproline, the precursor of collagen, in growing swine and found that there was a significant increase in the excretion rate of hydroxyproline following administration of the vitamin at levels up to 1 g daily for 32 days. Since 80 per cent of the hydroxyproline in urine is of bone origin, the raised hydroxyproline excretion was taken to indicate increased breakdown of bone collagen. This effect of vitamin C in mobilising bone minerals, may therefore result in a serious problem in growing children on daily vitamin supplements. At the same time, however, it is necessary to point out that there have been a number of reports suggesting that vitamin C in large doses may be beneficial in alleviating pain in bone disorders, such as Paget's disease of bone and secondary bone metastases (Section 5.4). Furthermore, Sifri, Kratzer and Norris (1977) in their study failed to notice any alterations in mineralisation of the bones of growing male chickens fed a diet containing 0.65 per cent vitamin C.

6.9 Infertility

There have been a few reports in the literature suggesting that vitamin C in large doses tends to favour infertility or abortion (Samborskaya and Ferdman, 1966). The inhibition of reproduction has also been found to be caused by administration of cAMP in female mice (Ryan and Coronel, 1969). Since vitamin C may increase the tissue level of cAMP (Section 3.2.2), it is possible that mega-intake of vitamin C may participate in arresting pregnancy by increasing tissue concentrations of cAMP. On the other hand, many workers have failed to observe such effects among their patients taking as much as 10 g of vitamin C daily for many years (Poser and Smith, 1972; Hoffer, 1973; Wilson and Loh, 1973).

Recently, Paul and Duttagupta (1978) investigated the effects of vitamin C in large doses (50 mg/day) on the reproductive organs in male rats fed either *ad libitum* or restricted diets. This study revealed that the restriction of diet alone reduced citric acid levels and the weight of reproductive organs and that vitamin C therapy improved these effects. On the other hand, vitamin C treatment of the *ad libitum* fed rats resulted in a reduction in the weight and citric acid content of the male reproductive glands. These findings seem to indicate that an excess of vitamin C reverses the adverse effects of diet restriction on the male reproductive glands, while it induces the adverse effects in the *ad libitum* fed animals.

6.10 Adaptation to High Vitamin C Intake

There is evidence that in some individuals the long-term administration of large doses of vitamin C leads to adaptation which might be responsible for the development of scurvy following sudden cessation of the extra vitamin intake (Schrauzer and Rhead, 1973). Cochrane (1975) reports two cases of infantile scurvy following maternal supplementation (400 mg/day) during pregnancy. This worker attributes this scurvy to systematic conditioning *in utero*. There have been a number of reports suggesting that similar effects could be produced in guinea pigs (Gordonoff, 1960; Norkus and Rosso, 1975).

In humans with adequate intakes of vitamin C, it has been shown that an initial increase in plasma vitamin C levels occurs following supplementary administration of 1–4 g/day of the vitamin, but within ten days the levels return to pre-treatment values in spite of the continuing high intake (Masek, Hruba and Novak, 1958; Spero and Anderson, 1973; Angel *et al.*, 1975). Upon stopping the extra vitamin C, abnormally low plasma levels of the vitamin appear to develop and then return to the original pre-treatment level again in about 14–21 days (Anderson, 1977). The evidence indicates that the rebound effect of sudden withdrawal of vitamin C may be attributed to increased metabolic utilisation or increased excretion of the vitamin in response to the increase in intake.

6.11 Effects on the Assay of Other Components in Biological Materials

It is known that the presence of vitamin C in the urine may give false positive results on tests for urinary sugar. The mechanisms by which the vitamin interferes with glucose estimations are believed to be mediated through the vitamin effects on the peroxide produced in glucose oxidase estimations, or the reduction of chemicals used in less specific tests for urine glucose (Free and Free, 1973). Such interference by vitamin C, however, may be avoided by either refraining from taking the vitamin on the day when the urine sample is obtained (Brandt,

Guyer and Banks, 1974) or using a separation technique such as chromatography.

Other common tests which have been reported to be affected by high dose vitamin C are those for blood in the stool, and estimations of serum transaminase, lactate dehydrogenase, bilirubin, uric acid and blood glucose (Siest *et al.*, 1978; Van Steirteghem, Robertson and Young, 1978). However, there are remarkably few effects of high plasma vitamin C concentrations on the analysis of other plasma components, and with the exception of blood glucose, most of the effects listed above are either slight or only occur at plasma concentrations of vitamin C which are extremely high and which would probably only arise following intravenous administration of large doses of the vitamin.

6.12 Conclusions

Evidence to date concerning the adverse effects of intakes of vitamin C which exceed the recommended intakes by large factors, appears to be contradictory. Further properly controlled studies are certainly warranted in order to clarify these conflicts. The nature of these studies should fall into three major categories: (1) the interaction of pharmacological doses of vitamin C or its metabolites with other nutrients and drugs; (2) the basic mechanisms underlying deleterious effects of large doses of the vitamin; (3) the delineation of the upper limit of safe vitamin intake in terms of both quantity and period of administration relative to the possible benefits derived from the dose. Until these studies are carried out, it is of paramount importance to take into consideration the reported adverse effects of megadoses of vitamin C, even if these are often either based on isolated cases or of a theoretical nature. Not only are large amounts of synthetic vitamin C readily obtainable without prescription, but more and more people are taking the vitamin in orthomolecular amounts, often along with prescribed drugs. Perhaps a slight risk of deleterious side effects of large doses of the vitamin is acceptable when administered for serious illness, such as malignant disease or immune deficiency conditions, but this is not so when the vitamin is taken in high doses for long periods by healthy or at least seemingly healthy individuals merely in the hope that it may protect against the common cold.

However, we must also emphasise that there is no evidence that, in those who are healthy, vitamin C intakes of up to 400 mg/day have any deleterious effects on health no matter how long they are maintained, or that 1—2 g taken daily, in an attempt to ameliorate the effects of the common cold, is harmful provided that the dose is only taken for a few days and that the individual is not receiving essential drug therapy such as anticonvulsive treatment or anticoagulants.

7 GENERAL CONCLUSIONS

Fifty years have passed since vitamin C was first identified and isolated. However, it is only in the last few years that our knowledge of the role of vitamin C in human metabolism has shown a significant advance. Here it is clear that vitamin C is involved in the hydroxylation (oxygenase) reactions required for the synthesis of collagen, carnitine and noradrenalin. Evidence suggests that relatively small quantities of vitamin C are needed in the tissues in order to fulfil many of these reactions, although optimal levels have not yet been established. In addition to these functions of vitamin C, there is evidence that pharmacological doses are of use in treating some conditions, particularly those involving depression of immunity, but it has not been adequately assessed how effective such doses will be in other diseases, such as atherosclerosis and malignancy, that have been reported to be prevented or treated by such intakes.

Our lack of knowledge of what tissue concentration is required for vitamin C to be maximally effective in carrying out its basic functions, is reflected in the differences which exist in recommended intakes from country to country (Table 7.1). Clearly intakes should be sufficiently high to prevent the development of scurvy and the 10 mg a day required to achieve this can easily be exceeded with an orange or a serving of green vegetables or new potatoes (not excessively cooked). Unfortunately, evidence suggests that a number of individuals in groups such as the elderly and the sick, fail to reach even these minimum intakes at certain times of the year and hence have vitamin C reserves equivalent to those found in clinical scurvy. In these populations the incidence of scurvy is surprisingly high. This is inappropriate and our first priority must be to ensure that at the very least this minimum intake is achieved throughout the year.

The suggestion that an optimum intake should be 60 mg a day, as this will prevent vitamin C reserves falling below the threshold at which hypovitaminosis C develops, is a more tenuous recommendation. However, this will certainly prevent the development of some of the early signs of scurvy such as behavioural change, muscle weakness and haemorrhage of small blood vessels and may indeed reduce the incidence of these clinical signs which are common in the elderly, the institutionalised and those with debilitating disease. An intake of 60 mg can

Table 7.1: Recommended Vitamin C Intakes in Some European Countries and in North America

Countries	Recommended Intake (mg/day)
Canada	30
Denmark	45
West Germany	75
Netherlands	50
Sweden	60
United Kingdom	30
United States	60
USSR	75

readily be obtained from the diet by consuming an average-sized orange or vitamin C-containing drink, plus a generous portion of both green vegetables and new potatoes each day. A list of foods rich in vitamin C is presented in Table 7.2. It must, however, be emphasised that storage of the fresh food for considreable periods or excessive cooking and hot storage will deplete the level of vitamin C considerably. Where increased intakes cannot be achieved by dietary means, because of anorexia or lack of motivation, then an appropriate vitamin preparation may be required.

Recommendations that attempt to improve the balance and quality of the diet as well as increasing vitamin C reserves are desirable because they will also increase levels of some of the other vitamins, such as folic acid, which are often depleted in association with low vitamin C reserves. It is also worth noting that vitamin C seems to have a sparing effect on other vitamins, such as thiamin.

The recommendation of 60 mg is for healthy individuals, but in disease and trauma there is an increased metabolism of vitamin C. However, in view of the fact that there is no evidence for intakes of up to 200 mg/day being toxic, we would not dissuade from doing so those individuals who wish to increase their intakes to this level as an insurance policy against any harmful effects of depleted tissue reserves. In short, for the healthy intakes of 60 mg per day are ideal, 200 mg will do no harm, although it may offer no advantage, whilst in some specific conditions, such as impaired immunity, hypercholesterolaemia and bone pain, pharmacological doses may be required. In such conditions the possible toxic effects of high intakes of vitamin C taken over many years are negligible compared with the reported beneficial effect on the disease process. Unfortunately, there is no conclusive

Table 7.2: A Selection of Foods Containing High Concentrations of Vitamin C

	Vitamin C mg/100 g
Freshly boiled vegetables:	
Broccoli	34
Brussels sprouts	40
Spring cabbage	25
Spinach	25
Cauliflower	20
New potatoes	18
Salad foods:	
Watercress	60
Tomatoes	20
Lettuce	15
Fruit:	
Blackcurrants (cooked)	140
Lemons	80
Strawberries	60
Oranges	38
Goosberries (cooked)	28
Apples (unpeeled)[a]	5–30

Cereals, cakes, milk products, eggs, nuts, confectionery, fish and meat (with the exception of offal and fish roes) contain little vitamin C.

Note: a. Depends on variety.
Source: Data taken from McCance and Widdowson (1978).

evidence yet that other conditions will respond to high dose vitamin C treatment.

It is clear that much work remains to be done. One of the areas in most need of investigation is the metabolism and breakdown of vitamin C, as such knowledge will aid our understanding of any changes that occur in our requirement for the vitamin during disease. Vitamin researchers have always been handicapped by the difficulty in carrying out conventional balance studies where the rate of utilisation of the vitamin can be assessed. The main problem is the difficulty in measuring the catabolic products of vitamin metabolism which escape in the urine, stool and sweat. Not only are some of these products of vitamin C metabolism undetectable by the conventional assay procedures, but some have yet to be identified. With better techniques, which include the use of isotopes, mass spectrometry, high performance liquid chromatography and isotacophoresis, the identification and measurement of the breakdown products of vitamin C should become feasible.

Other areas that require further study are: the effects on health of hypovitaminosis C and the contribution, if any, that low vitamin C reserves make to degenerative disease; appropriately controlled clinical trials in conditions where claims have been made for a pharmacological effect of the vitamin; the metabolic interrelationships of different vitamins and the possible additive detrimental effects of marginal depletion of several vitamins. It may be that such studies will eventually reveal that vitamin C is only required at the minimal intake needed to prevent overt scurvy, which some individuals still fail to acquire. However, current evidence suggests that this is not the case and that higher intakes, which many individuals fail to achieve, will be required to maintain health and prevent degenerative change. Because both hypovitaminosis C and the associated degenerative changes are common, it is necessary to proceed with all haste to prove or refute a cause-and-effect relationship.

REFERENCES

Aarts, E. M. (1968). *Biochem. Pharma.*, *17*, 327

Abbasy, M. A., Harris, L. J. and Ellman, P. (1937). *Lancet, 2*, 181

Abt, A. F. and Farmer, C. J. (1938). *J. Am. Med. Assoc., 8*, 1555

Akerfeldt, S. (1957). *Science, 125*, 117

Allen, R. J. L., Brook, M. and Broadbent, S. R. (1968). *Brit. J. Nutr., 22*, 555

Anah, C. O., Jarike, L. N. and Baig, H. A. (1980). *Trop. Geogr. Med., 32*, 132

Anderson, R. (1979). *S. Afr. Med. J., 56*, 401

—— (1981). In *Vitamin C*, ed. Counsell, J. and Hornig, D. Applied Science Pub. Ltd, London

Anderson, R. and Dittrich, O. C. (1979). *S. Afr. Med. J., 56*, 476

Anderson, R., Oosthuizen, R. and Gatner, E. M. S. (1979). *S. Afr. Med. J., 56*, 511

Anderson, R., Oosthuizen, R., Maritz, R., Theron, A. and Van Rensburg, A. J. (1980). *Am. J. Clin. Nutr., 33*, 21

Anderson, R. and Theron, A. (1979a). *S. Afr. Med. J., 56*, 394

—— (1979b). *S. Afr. Med. J., 56*, 429

Anderson, T. W. (1977). *Acta. Vitam. Enzymologica, 31*, 43

Anderson, T. W., Beaton, G. H., Corey, P. N. and Spero, L. (1975). *Can. Med. Assoc. J., 112*, 823

Anderson, T. W., Reid, D. B. W. and Beaton, G. H. (1972). *Can. Med. Assoc. J., 107*, 503

Andrews, J., Brook, M. and Allen, M. A. (1966). *Geront. Clin., 8*, 257

Andrews, J., Letcher, M. and Brook, M. (1969). *Br. Med. J., 2*, 416

Angel, J., Alfred, B., Leichter, J., Lee, M. and Marchaut, L. (1975). *Int. J. Vitam. & Nutr. Res., 45*, 237

Anson, G. (1748). In *A Voyage Round the World*, compiled by Richard Walter. John & Paul Knapton, London

Archer, M. C., Tannenbaum, S. R., Fan, T. Y. and Weisman, M. (1975). *J. Natn. Cancer Inst., 54*, 1203

Arthur, G., Monro, J. A., Poore, P., Rilwan, W. B., Murphy, E. and La, C. (1967). *Br. Med. J., 1*, 732

Atkins, G. L., Dean, B. M., Griffin, W. J., Scowen, E. F. and Watts, R. W. E. (1963). *Lancet, 2*, 1096

Atkinson, J. P., Weiss, A., Ito, M., Kelly, J. and Parker, C. W. (1979).

J. Cyclic Nucleotide Res., *5*, 107

Attwood, E. C., Robey, E. D., Ross, J., Bradley, F. and Kramer, J. J. (1974). *Clinica Chim. Acta, 54*, 95

Avigliano, L., Rotilio, G., Urbanelli, S., Mondovi, B. and Agro, A. F. (1978). *Archs. Biochem. Biophys., 185*, 419

Babior, B. M. (1977). In *EMBO Workshop on Superoxide and Super-oxide Dismutase*, ed. Michelson, A. M., McCord, J. M. and Fridovich, I., p. 271. Academic Press, London and New York

Baird, I. M., Hughes, R. E., Wilson, H. K., Davies, J. E. W. and Howard, A. N. (1979). *Am. J. Clin. Nutr., 32*, 1686

Baker, E. M. (1967). *Am. J. Clin. Nutr., 20*, 583

Baker, E. M., Hodges, R. E., Hood, J., Sauberlich, H. E. and March, S. C. (1969). *Am. J. Clin. Nutr., 22*, 549

Baker, E. M., Hodges, R. E., Hood, J., Sauberlich, H. E., March, S. C. and Canham, J. E. (1971). *Am. J. Clin. Nutr., 24*, 444

Baker, E. M., Saari, J. C. and Tolbert, B. M. (1966). *Am. J. Clin. Nutr., 19*, 371

Baker, E. M., Sauberlich, H. E., Wolfskill, S. J., Wallace, W. T. and Dean, E. E. (1962). *Proc. Soc. Expt. Biol. Med., 109*, 737

Banerjee, S. and Nandy, N. (1970). *Proc. Soc. Expt. Biol. Med., 133*, 151

Barkhan, P. and Howard, A. N. (1958). *Biochem. J., 70*, 163

Barnes, M. J. (1975). *Ann. N.Y. Acad. Sci., 258*, 264

Barnes, M. J. and Kodicek, E. (1972). *Vitam. Horm., 30*, 1

Bartlett, M. K., Jones, C. M. and Ryan, A. E. (1940). *Ann. Surg., 111*, 1
―― (1942). *New.Eng. J. Med., 226*, 474

Bartley, W., Krebs, H. A. and O'Brien, J. R. P. (1953). *Spec. Rep. Ser. Med. Res. Coun.*, no. 280. HMSO, London

Barton, G. M. G., Laing, J. E. and Barisoni, D. (1972). *Int. J. Vitam. & Nutr. Res., 42*, 524

Basu, T. K. (1977). *Chemico-Biol. Interactions, 16*, 247
―― (1979). *Int. J. Vitam. & Nutr. Res.*, Suppl. no. 19, 95
―― (1980). In *Clinical Implications of Drug Use*, ed. Basu, T. K., vol. 1, p. 11. CRC Press, Florida

Basu, T. K. and Dickerson, J. W. T. (1974). *Chemico-Biol. Interactions, 8*, 193

Basu, T. K., Donaldson, D. and Williams, D. C. (1974). *Oncology, 30*, 197

Basu, T. K., Jenner, M. and Williams, D. C. (1976). *Nutr. Metabol., 20*, 425

Basu, T. K., Raven, R. W., Dickerson, J. W. T. and Williams, D. C.

(1974). *Eur. J. Cancer, 10*, 507

Basu, T. K., Smethurst, M., Gillett, M. B., Donaldson, D., Jordan, S. J., Williams, D. C. and Hicklin, J. A. (1978). *Acta Vitam. Enzymologica, 32*, 45

Bates, C. J. (1977). *Clin. Sci., 52*, 535

Bates, C. J., Flemming, M., Paul, A. A., Black, A. E. and Mandal, A. R. (1980). *Age & Ageing, 9*, 1

Bates, C. J., Mandal, A. R. and Cole, T. J. (1977). *Lancet, 2*, 611

Bates, C. J., Rutishauser, I. H. E., Black, A. E., Paul, A. A., Mandal, A. R. and Patnaik, B. K. (1979). *Br. J. Nutr., 42*, 43

Bates, J. F., Hughes, R. E. and Hurley, R. J. (1972). *Archs. Oral. Biol., 17*, 1017

Beattie, A. D. and Sherlock, S. (1976). *Gut, 17*, 571

Beisel, W. R., Herman, Y. F., Sauberlich, H. E., Herman, R. E., Bartelloni, P. J. and Canham, J. E. (1972). *Am. J. Clin. Nutr., 25*, 1165

Benade, L., Howard, T. and Burk, D. (1969). *Oncology, 23*, 33

Benassi, C. A., Perissiotto, B. and Allegri, G. (1963). *Clinica Chim. Acta, 8*, 822

Bessey, O. A. (1938). *J. Biol. Chem., 126*, 771

Bingol, A., Altay, C., Say, B. and Donmez, S. (1975). *J. Pediat., 86*, 902

Bishun, N., Basu, T. K., Metcalfe, S. and Williams, D. C. (1978). *Oncology, 35*, 160

Bjorkhem, I. and Kallner, A. (1976). *J. Lipid Res., 17*, 360

Bjorksten, J. (1979). *Rejuvenation, 2*, 33

BMJ, Leading Article (1977). *Br. Med. J., 1*, 735

Boehringer Mannheim GMBH (1980). *Methods of Enzymatic Food Analysis.* BCL, Lewes

Bonjour, J. P. (1979). *Int. J. Vitam. & Nutr. Res., 49*, 434

Booth, J. B. and Todd, G. B. (1972). *Geriatrics, 27*, 130

Bordia, A. (1980). *Atherosclerosis, 35*, 181

Bordia, A., Paliwal, D. K., Jain, K. and Kothari, L. K. (1978). *Atherosclerosis, 30*, 351

Bouhuys, A., Hunt, V. R., Kim, B. M. and Zapletal, A. (1969). *J. Clin. Invest., 48*, 1159

Bourne, G. (1938). *Br. Med. J., 1*, 560

Bourne, G. H. (1946). *Proc. Nutr. Soc., 4*, 204

Bowers, E. F. and Kubik, M. M. (1965). *Br. J. Clin. Pract., 19*, 141

Boxer, L. A., Albertini, D. F., Baehner, R. L. and Oliver, J. M. (1979). *Br. J. Haemat., 43*, 207

Boyland, E. and Grover, P. L. (1961). *Biochem. J., 81*, 163

Bram, S., Froussard, P., Guichard, M., Jasmin, C., Augery, Y., Sinoussi-Barre, F. and Wray, W. (1980). *Nature, 284,* 629

Brandt, R., Guyer, K. E. and Banks, W. L., Jr. (1974). *Clinica Chim. Acta, 51,* 103

Briggs, M. H. and Briggs, M. (1973). *Lancet, 1,* 998

Briggs, M. H., Gracia-Webb, P. and Davies, P. (1973). *Lancet, 2,* 201

Brin, M. (1980). *Am. J. Clin. Nutr., 33,* 169

Brocklehurst, J. C., Griffiths, L. L., Taylor, G. F., Marks, J., Scott, D. L. and Blackley, J. (1968). *Geront. Clin., 10,* 309

Bronte-Stewart, B., Roberts, B. and Wells, U. M. (1963). *Br. J. Nutr., 17,* 61

Brook, M. and Grimshaw, J. J. (1968). *Am. J. Clin. Nutr., 21,* 1254

Brown, M. S. and Goldstein, J. L. (1974). *Science, 185,* 61

Brown, R. G., Sharma, V. D. and Young, L. G. (1971). *Can. J. Anim. Sci., 51,* 439

Burke, B. S. (1947). *J. Am. Diet. Ass., 23,* 1041

Burns, J. J. (1957). *J. Am. Chem. Soc., 74,* 1257

Burr, M. L., Elwood, P. C., Hole, D. J., Hurley, R. J. and Hughes, R. E. (1974). *Am. J. Clin. Nutr., 27,* 144

Busieno, L. (1949). *Boll. Soc. Ital. Biol. Sper., 25,* 274

Calder, J. H., Curtis, R. C. and Fore, H. (1963). *Lancet, 1,* 556

Cameron, E. (1975). *Br. J. Hosp. Med., 13,* 511

Cameron, E. and Baird, G. M. (1973). *IRCS Med. Sci., 8,* 38

Cameron, E. and Campbell, A. (1974). *Chemico-Biol. Interactions, 9,* 285

Cameron, E. and Pauling, L. (1976). *Proc. Natl. Acad. Sci., 73,* 3865
—— (1978). *Proc. Natl. Acad. Sci., 75,* 4538

Cameron, E., Pauling, L. and Leibovitz, B. (1979). *Cancer Res., 39,* 663

Campbell, G. D., Steinberg, M. H. and Bower, J. D. (1975). *Ann. Intern. Med., 82,* 810

Candlish, J. K. and Tristram, G. R. (1963). *Biochim. Biophys. Acta, 78,* 289

Carneiro, J. and Fava de Moraes, F. (1965). *Arch. Oral Biol., 10,* 833

Chalmers, T. C. (1975). *Am. J. Med., 58,* 532

Charkrabarti, B. and Banerjee, S. (1955). *Proc. Soc. Expt. Biol. Med., 88,* 581

Chatterjee, I. B., Majumder, A. K., Nandi, B. K. and Subramanian, N. (1975). *Ann. N.Y. Acad. Sci., 258,* 24

Cheraskin, E. and Ringsdorf, W. M. Jr. (1979). *J. Electrocardiol., 12,* 441

Chope, H. D. (1954). *Calif. Med., 81,* 335

Chope, H. D. and Dray, S. (1951). *Calif. Med., 74*, 105

Chu, T. M. and Slaunwhite, W. R. Jr. (1968). *Steroids, 12*, 309

Clemetson, C. A. B. (1979). *Med. Hypotheses, 5*, 825

Cochrane, W. A. (1965). *Can. Med. Assoc. J., 93*, 893

Conney, A. H., Bray, G. A., Evans, C. and Burns, J. J. (1961). *Ann. N.Y. Acad. Sci., 92*, 126

Conney, A. H. and Burns, J. J. (1959). *Nature, 184*, 363

Coon, W. W. (1962). *Surgery Gynec. Obstet., 115*, 522

Cormia, F. E. (1941). *J. Invest. Derm., 4*, 81

Coulehan, J. L. (1979). *Postgrad. Med., 66*, 153

Coulehan, J. L., Eberhard, S., Kapner, L. and Taylor, F. (1976). *New Eng. J. Med., 295*, 973

Coulehan, J. L., Reisinger, K. S., Rogers, K. D. and Bradley, D. W. (1974). *New Eng. J. Med., 290*, 6

Cowan, A. (1976). *Ir. J. Med. Sci., 145*, 273

Cox, E. V. (1968). *Vitam. Horm., 26*, 635

Cramer, H. and Schultz, J. (1977). *Cyclic 3',5-Nucleotides. Mechanism of Action.* Wiley-Interscience Publications, London

Crandon, J. H., Landau, B., Mikal, S., Balmanno, J., Jefferson, M. and Mahoney, N. (1958). *New Eng. J. Med., 258*, 105

Crandon, J. H., Lennihan, R., Mikal, S. and Reif, A. E. (1961). *Ann. N.Y. Acad. Sci., 92*, 246

Crandon, J. H. and Lund, C. C. (1940). *New Eng. J. Med., 222*, 748

Crandon, J. H., Lund, C. C. and Dill, D. B. (1940). *New Eng. J. Med., 223*, 353

Crawford, G. P. M., Warlow, C. P., Bennett, B., Dawson, A. A., Douglas, A. S., Kerridge, D. F. and Ogston, D. (1975). *Atherosclerosis, 21*, 451

Creagan, E. T., Moertel, G. G., O'Fallon, J. R., Schutt, A. J., O'Connell, M. J., Rubin, J. and Fryfar, S. (1979). *New Eng. J. Med., 301*, 687

Cuschieri, C. (1973). *Br. J. Surg., 60*, 800

Cutforth, R. H. (1958). *Lancet, 1*, 454

Dallegri, F., Lanzi, G. and Patrone, F. (1980). *Int. Archs. Allergy Appl. Immun., 61*, 40

Davidson, S., Passmore, R. and Brock, J. F. (1972). *Human Nutrition and Dietetics*, 5th edn, p. 176. E. S. Livingstone Ltd, Edinburgh and London

Davies, J. D. G. and Newson, J. (1974). *Am. J. Clin. Nutr., 27*, 1039

Davies, J. E. W., Hughes, R. E., Jones, E., Reed, S. E., Craig, J. W. and Tyrrell, D. A. J. (1979). *Biochem. Med., 21*, 78

Dawson, K. P. and Duncan, A. (1975). *Br. J. Nutr., 33*, 315

Dawson, W. and West, G. B. (1965). *J. Pharm. Pharmac.*, *17*, 595

Day, B. R., Williams, D. R. and Marsh, C. A. (1979). *Clin. Biochem.*, *12*, 22

Deana, R., Bharaj, B. S., Verjee, Z. H. and Galzigna, L. (1975). *Int. J. Vitam. & Nutr. Res.*, *45*, 175

De Cosse, J. J., Adams, M. B., Kuzma, J. F., Logerfo, P. and Condon, R. E. (1975). *Surgery*, *78*, 608

De Fabro, S. P. (1967). *C.R. Seanc. Soc. Biol.*, *162*, 284

Degkwitz, E., Walsch, S., Dubberstein, M. and Winter, J. (1975). *Ann. N.Y. Acad. Sci.*, *258*, 201

Delp, M. (1941). *J. Kans. Med. Soc.*, *42*, 519

Denson, K. W. and Bowers, E. F. (1961). *Clin. Sci.*, *21*, 157

Department of Health and Social Security. (1969). *Rep. Publ. Hlth. Med. Subj.*, no. 120. HMSO, London

Dewhurst, F. and Kitchen, D. A. (1973). *Biochem. Pharmac.*, *22*, 789

Dice, J. F. and Daniel, C. W. (1973). *J. Int. Res. Commun. Med. Sci.*, *1*, 41

Disselduff, M. M., Murphy, E. and La, C. (1968). In *Vitamins in the Elderly*, ed. Exton-Smith, A. N. and Scott, D. L., p. 60. John Wright & Sons Ltd, Bristol

Dunnigan, M. G. and Harland, W. A. (1970). *Lancet*, *2*, 793

Dutra de Oliveira, J. E., Pearson, W. N. and Darby, W. I. (1959). *Am. J. Clin. Nutr.*, *7*, 630

Eddy, T. P. (1968). In *Vitamins in the Elderly*, ed. Exton-Smith, A. N. and Scott, D. L., p. 86. John Wright and Sons Ltd, Bristol

—— (1972). *Br. J. Nutr.*, *27*, 537

Eddy, T. P. and Taylor, G. F. (1977). *Age & Ageing*, *6*, 6

Edgar, J. A. (1970). *Nature*, *227*, 24

Elsas, L. J., Hollins, B. and Pinnell, S. R. (1974). *Am. J. Hum. Genet.*, *26*, 28

Elwood, P. C., Hughes, R. E. and Hurley, R. J. (1970). *Lancet*, *2*, 1197

Evans, R. M., Currie, L. and Campbell, A. (1980). *Ann. Clin. Biochem.*, *17*, 252

Exton-Smith, A. N. (1980). Report on Health and Social Subjects No. 16. Department of Health and Social Security, HMSO, London

Faulkner, J. M. and Taylor, F. H. L. (1937). *Ann. Intern. Med.*, *10*, 1867

Feetam, C. L., Leach, R. H. and Meynell, M. J. (1975). *Toxicol. Appl. Pharmacol.*, *31*, 544

Fiddler, W., Pensabene, J. W., Piotrowski, E. G., Doerr, R. C. and Wassherman, J. (1973). *J. Food. Sci.*, *38*, 1084

Fielding, A. M. and Hughes, R. E. (1975). *Experientia, 31*, 1394

Finkle, P. (1937). *J. Clin. Invest., 16*, 587

Food and Nutrition Board, National Research Council. (1974). *Recommended Dietary Allowances*, 8th edn. National Academy of Sciences, Washington DC

—— (1980). *Recommended Dietary Allowances*, 9th edn. National Academy of Sciences, Washington DC

Fox, F. W., Dangerfield, L. F., Gottlich, S. F. and Jokl, E. (1940). *Br. Med. J., 2*, 143

Free, H. M. and Free, A. H. (1973). *Clin. Chem., 19*, 662

Friedman, G. D., Siegelaub, A. B., Seltzer, C. C., Feldman, R. and Collen, M. F. (1973). *Archs. Envir. Hlth., 26*, 137

Friedman, G. J., Sherry, S. and Ralli, E. P. (1940). *J. Clin. Invest., 19*, 685

Friend, D. G. and Marquis, H. H. (1938). *Am. J. Syph. Gonorrhea Vener. Dis., 22*, 239

Fujinami, T., Okado, K., Senda, K., Sugimura, M. and Kishikawa, M. (1971). *Jap. Circul. J., 35*, 1559

Gallin, J. I., Elin, R. J., Hubert, R. T., Fauci, A. S., Kaliner, M. A. and Wolff, S. M. (1979). *Blood, 53*, 226

Garry, P. J. and Owen, G. M. (1968). In *Technicon Symposia, 1*, 507

Geoly, K. L. and Diamond, L. H. (1980). *Ann. Intern. Med., 93*, 511

Geriatrics, Editorial (1978). New Frontiers of Research. *Geriatrics, 33*, 91

Gerson, C. D. (1975). *Ann. N.Y. Acad. Sci., 258*, 483

Gibson, S. L. M., Moore, F. M. L. and Goldberg, A. (1966). *Br. Med. J., 1*, 1152

Ginter, E. (1972). *Lancet, 1*, 1233

—— (1973). *Science, 179*, 702

—— (1975). *Ann. N.Y. Acad. Sci., 258*, 410

—— (1976). *New Eng. J. Med., 294*, 559

—— (1978). *Adv. Lipid Res., 16*, 167

—— (1979a). *Wld. Rev. Nutr. Diet., 33*, 104

—— (1979b). *Lancet, 2*, 958

—— (1979c). *Am. J. Clin. Nutr., 32*, 511

Ginter, E., Babala, J. and Cerven, J. (1969). *J. Atheroscler. Res., 10*, 341

Ginter, E., Bobek, P., Babala, J., Jakubovsky, J., Zaviacic, M. and Lojda, Z. (1979). In *Vitamin C — Recent Advances and Aspects in Virus Diseases, Cancer and in Lipid Metabolism*, ed. Hanck, A. and Ritzel, G., p. 55. Hans Huber, Bern

Ginter, E., Bobek, P., Kopec, Z., Ovecka, M. and Cerey, K. (1967). *Z. Versuchstierk., 9*, 228

Ginter, E., Kajaba, I. and Nizner, O. (1970). *Nutr. Metabolism, 12*, 76

Ginter, E., Ondreicka, R., Bobek, P. and Simko, V. (1969). *J. Nutr., 99*, 261

Ginter, E., Zdichynec, B., Holzerova, O., Ticha, E., Kobza, R., Koziakova, M., Cerna, O., Ozdin, L., Hruba, F., Novakova, V., Sasko, E. and Gaher, M. (1978). *Int. J. Vitam. & Nutr. Res., 48*, 368

Glew, G., Hill, M. A. and Millross, J. (1971). In *Proceedings of University of Nottingham Residential Seminar on Vitamins*, ed. Mendel, G. H. and Stein, S. R., p. 81. Churchill Livingstone, Edinburgh

Glickman, I. (1948a). *J. Dent. Res., 27*, 9

——— (1948b). *J. Dent. Res., 27*, 201

Goetzl, E. J., Wasserman, S. I., Gigli, I. and Austen, F. K. (1974). *J. Clin. Invest., 53*, 813

Goldberg, A. (1963). *Q. J. Med., 32* (New Series), 51

Goldsmith, G. A. (1961). *Ann. N.Y. Acad. Sci., 92*, 230

——— (1971). *J. Am. Med. Assoc., 216*, 216

Gordonoff, T. (1960). *Schweiz. Med. Wschr., 90*, 726

Gould, B. S. (1963). *Int. Rev. Cytol., 15*, 301

Griffiths, L. L. (1968). In *Vitamins in the Elderly*, ed. Exton-Smith, A. N. and Scott, D. L., p. 34. John Wright & Sons Ltd, Bristol

Griffiths, L. L., Brocklehurst, J. C., Scott, D. L., Marks, J. and Blackley, J. (1967). *Geront. Clin., 9*, 1

Guttemplan, J. B. (1977). *Nature, 268*, 368

Hagtvet, J. (1945). *Nord. Med., 28*, 2335

Hammerstroem, L. (1966). *Acta Physiol. Scand., 70*, 1

Hanck, A. and Weiser, H. (1977). In *Re-evaluation of Vitamin C*, ed. Hanck, A. and Ritzel, G., p. 67. Verlag, Hans Huber, Bern, Stuttgart and Wein

Hanck, L. V., Jansen, C. R. and Schmaeler, M. (1974). *Biochem. Med., 9*, 1974

Harris, L. J. and Olliver, M. (1943). *Lancet, 1*, 454

Hayaishi, O., Nozaki, M. and Abbott, M. T. (1975). In *The Enzymes*, ed. Boyer, P. D., Vol. XII, Part B, p. 119. Academic Press, London and New York

Hellman, L. and Burns, J. J. (1958). *J. Biol. Chem., 230*, 923

Henry, R. J., Cannon, D. C. and Winkleman, J. W. (1974). *Clinical Chemistry Principles and Technics*, 2nd edn, p. 1394. Harper and Row, London and New York

Herbert, V. and Jacob, E. (1974). *J. Am. Med. Assoc., 230*, 241

Herbert, V., Jacob, E., Wong, K. T. J., Scott, J. and Pfeffer, R. D. (1978). *Am. J. Clin. Nutr., 31*, 253

Herjanic, M. and Moss-Herjanic, B. L. (1967). *J. Schizophrenia, 1*, 257

Hill, G. L., Pickford, I., Young, G. A., Schorah, C. J., Blackett, R. L., Burkinshaw, L., Warren, J. V. and Morgan, D. B. (1977). *Lancet, 1*, 689

Hines, J. D. (1975). *J. Am. Med. Assoc., 234*, 24

Hodges, R. E., Hood, J., Canham, J. E., Sauberlich, H. E. and Baker, E. M. (1971). *Am. J. Clin. Nutr., 24*, 432

Hoffer, A. (1973). *Lancet, 2*, 1146

Hoffer, A. and Osmond, H. (1967). *Dis. Nerv. Syst., 24*, 273

Hogenkamp, H. P. C. (1980). *Am. J. Clin. Nutr., 33*, 1

Holmes, H. N. (1943). *J. Sth. Med. Ass., 105*, 393

Holmes, H. N. and Alexander, W. (1942). *Science, 96*, 497

Hornig, D. (1975). *Ann. N.Y. Acad. Sci., 258*, 103

——— (1977). *Acta Vitam. Enzymologica, 31*, 9

Hornig, D., Vulleumier, J. P. and Hartmann, D. (1980). *Int. J. Vitam. & Nutr. Res., 50*, 309

Hornig, D. and Weiser, H. (1976). *Experientia, 32*, 687

Hornig, D., Weiser, H., Weber, F. and Wiss, O. (1973). *Int. J. Vitam. & Nutr. Res., 43*, 28

Horrobin, D. F., Oka, M. and Manku, M. S. (1979). *Med. Hypotheses, 5*, 849

Houston, J. B. and Levy, G. (1975). *Nature, 255*, 78

Howald, H. and Segessar, B. (1975). *Ann. N.Y. Acad. Sci., 258*, 458

Howard, A. N. and Constable, B. J. (1966). *Clinica Chim. Acta, 13*, 387

Hubmann, B., Monnier, D. and Roth, M. (1969). *Clinica Chim. Acta, 25*, 161

Hughes, R. E. (1964). *Analyst, 89*, 618

Hughes, R. E., Hurley, R. J. and Jones, E. (1980). *Br. J. Nutr., 43*, 385

Hughes, R. E. and Williams, N. (1978). *Digestion, 17*, 272

Hulse, J. D., Ellis, S. R. and Henderson, L. M. (1978). *J. Biol. Chem., 253*, 1654

Hume, R., Johnstone, J. M. S. and Weyers, E. (1972). *J. Am. Med. Assoc., 219*, 1479

Hume, R. and Weyers, E. (1973). *Scott. Med. J., 18*, 3

Hume, R., Weyers, E., Rowan, T., Reid, D. S. and Hillis, W. S. (1972). *Br. Heart J., 34*, 238

Hunter, T. and Rajan, K. T. (1971). *Paraplegia, 8*, 211

Iggo, B., Owen, J. A. and Stewart, C. P. (1956). *Clinica Chim. Acta, 1*, 167

Ikonopisov, R. L. (1972). In *Melanoma and Skin Cancer*, ed. McCarthy, W. H., p. 223. International Union Against Cancer, Sydney

Ingalls, T. H. and Warren, H. A. (1937). *New Eng. J. Med., 217*, 443

Irvin, T. T., Chattopadhyay, D. K. and Smythe, A. (1978). *Surgery Gynec. Obstet., 147*, 49

Irwin, M. I. and Hutchins, B. K. (1976). *J. Nutr., 106*, 821

Johnston, R. B. and Lehmeyer, J. E. (1977). In *EMBO Workshop on Superoxide and Superoxide Dismutase*, ed. Michelson, A. M., McCord, J. M. and Fridovich, I., p. 291. Academic Press, London and New York

Kajaba, A. B. (1968). *Rev. Czech. Med., 14*, 180

Kakar, S. C., Wilson, C. W. M. and Bell, J. N. (1975). *Ir. J. Med. Sci., 144*, 227

Kallner, A., Hartmann, D. and Hornig, D. (1977). *Nutr. Metabolism, 21*, 31

—— (1979). *Am. J. Clin. Nutr., 32*, 530

Kamm, J. J., Dashman, T., Conney, A. H. and Burns, J. J. (1973). *Proc. Natl. Acad. Sci., 70*, 747

Kanis, J. A., Horn, D. B., Scott, R. D. M. and Strong, J. A. (1974). *Br. Med. J., 3*, 727

Kataria, M. S. and Rao, D. B. (1965). *Geront. Clin., 7*, 189

Kaufman, S. and Friedman, S. (1965). *Pharmacol. Rev., 17*, 71

Keith, R. E. and Driskell, J. A. (1980). *Nutr. Rep. Int., 21*, 907

Kelleher, J. (1979). In *The Importance of Vitamins to Human Health*, ed. Taylor, T. G., p. 139. MTP Press, Lancaster

Kinsman, R. A. and Hood, J. (1971). *Am. J. Clin. Nutr., 24*, 455

Kirk, J. E. (1962). *Vitam. Horm., 20*, 67

Kirk, J. E. and Chieffi, M. (1953a). *J. Geront,, 8*, 301

—— (1953b). *J. Geront., 8*, 305

Klasson, D. H. (1951). *N.Y. St. J. Med., 51*, 2388

Klenner, F. R. (1971). *J. Applied Nutr., 23*, 61

Knox, E. G. (1973). *Lancet, 1*, 1465

Kotzé, J. P. and Spies, J. H. (1976). *S. Afr. Med. J., 50*, 1760

Krasner, N. and Dymock, I. W. (1974). *Br. J. Cancer, 30*, 142

Kritchevsky, D., Tepper, S. A. and Story, J. A. (1973). *Lipids, 8*, 482

Kubler, W. and Gehler, J. (1970). *Int. J. Vitam. & Nutr. Res., 40*, 442

Kuenzig, W., Avenia, R. and Kamm, J. J. (1974). *J. Nutr., 104*, 952

Kum-Tatt, L. and Leong, P. C. (1964). *Clin. Chem., 10*, 575

Kurz, D. and Eyring, E. J. (1974). *Pediatrics, 54*, 56

Kyaw, A. (1978). *Clinica Chim. Acta, 86*, 153

La Du, B. N. and Zannoni, V. G. (1961). *Ann. N.Y. Acad. Sci., 92*, 175

Lamden, M. P. (1971). *New Eng. J. Med., 284*, 336
Lamden, M. P. and Chrystowski, G. A. (1954). *Proc. Soc. Expt. Biol. Med., 85*, 190
Lamden, M. P. and Schweiker, C. E. (1955). *Fedn. Proc., 14*, 439
Lawrence, J. C., Xabregas, A., Gray, L. and Ham, J. M. (1977). *Br. J. Surg., 64*, 777
Leevy, C. M., Thompson, A. and Baker, H. (1970). *Am. J. Clin. Nutr., 23*, 493
Lehninger, A. L. (1975). *Biochemistry*, 2nd edn, p. 502. Worth, New York
Lester, D., Buccino, R. and Bizzocco, D. (1960). *J. Nutr., 70*, 278
Levine, S. Z. (1947). *Harvey Lect., 42*, 303
Lewin, S. (1976). *Vitamin C: Its Molecular Biology and Medical Potential*. Academic Press, London and New York
Linaker, B. D. (1979). *Postgrad. Med. J., 55*, 26
Lind, J. (1753). *A Treatise of the Scurvy*. Sands, Murray and Cochrane, Edinburgh. Reprinted, ed. Stewart, C. P. and Guthrie, D., Edinburgh University Press, Edinburgh, 1953
Lloyd, J. V., Davis, P. S., Emery, H. and Lander, H. (1972). *J. Clin. Path., 25*, 478
Logue, T. and Frommer, D. (1980). *Aust. & N.Z. J. Med., 10*, 588
Loh, H. S. (1971). *Int. J. Vitam. & Nutr. Res., 42*, 80
Losert, W., Vetter, H. and Wendt, H. (1980). *Arzneimittel-Forsch., 30–1*, 21
Lowry, O. H., Bessey, O. A., Brock, M. J. and Lopez, J. A. (1946). *J. Biol. Chem., 166*, 111
Lowry, O. H., Bessey, O. A. and Burch, H. P. (1952). *Proc. Soc. Expt. Biol. Med., 80*, 361
Lugg, J. W. H. (1942). *Aust. J. Exp. Biol. Med. Sci., 20*, 273
Lund, C. C. (1939). *New Eng. J. Med., 221*, 121
Lynch, S. R., Sefel, H. C., Torrance, J. D., Charlton, R. W. and Bothwell, T. H. (1967). *Am. J. Clin. Nutr., 20*, 641
Machtey, I., Syrkis, I. and Fried, M. (1975). *Clinica Chim. Acta, 62*, 149
Maciennan, W. J. and Hamilton, J. C. (1976). *Age and Ageing, 5*, 43
Malamud, D. and Kroll, Y. (1980). *Proc. Soc. Expt. Biol. Med., 164*, 534
Mann, G. V. and Newton, P. (1975). *Ann. N.Y. Acad. Sci., 258*, 243
Manzella, J. P. and Roberts, N. J. (1979). *J. Immun., 123*, 1940
Martin, G. J. and Heise, F. H. (1937–38). *Am. J. Dig. Dis., 4*, 368
Martin, M. P., Bridgforth, E., McGanity, W. J. and Darby, W. J. (1957). *J. Nutr., 62*, 201

Masek, J., Hruba, F. and Novak, M. (1958). *Ernährungsforschung, 3*, 425

Mathen, V. I., Baker, S. J., Sood, S. K., Ramachandran, K. and Ramalingaswami, V. (1979). *Br. J. Nutr., 42*, 391

Mayersohn, M. (1972). *Eur. J. Pharmacol., 19*, 140

Maynwaringe, E. (1672). *A Treatise of the Scurvy*, p. 43. London

McCance, R. A. and Widdowson, E. M. (1960). *The Composition of Foods, Spec. Rep. Ser. Med. Res. Coun.*, no. 297. HMSO: London
—— (1978). *The Composition of Foods*. Revised by Paul, A. A. and Southgate, D. A. T., 4th edn. *Spec. Rep. Ser. Med. Res. Coun.*, no. 297. HMSO, London

McClean, H. E., Dodds, P. M., Abernetly, M. H., Stewart, A. W. and Beaven, D. W. (1976). *N.Z. Med. J., 83*, 226

McClean, H. E., Dodds, P. M. and Stewart, A. W. (1976). *N.Z. Med. J., 84*, 345

McCraw, A. and Sim, A. K. (1969). *Clinica Chim. Acta, 25*, 286

McGinn, F. P. and Hamilton, J. C. (1976). *Br. J. Surg., 63*, 505

McKusick, V. A. (1974). *Mendelian Inheritance in Man*, 4th edn, p. 412. Johns Hopkins University Press, Baltimore

Mengel, C. E. and Greene, H. L. (1976). *Ann. Intern. Med., 84*, 490

Migliozzi, J. A. (1977). *Br. J. Cancer, 35*, 448

Miller, J. Z., Nance, W. E., Norton, J. A., Wolen, R. L., Griffith, R. S. and Rose, R. J. (1977). *J. Am. Med. Assoc., 237*, 248

Miller, R. L., Elsas, L. J. and Priest, R. E. (1979). *J. Invest. Derm., 72*, 241

Millross, J., Speht, A., Holdsworth, K. and Glew, G. (1973). *The Utilisation of the Cook-Freeze System for School Meals*. Maney & Son, Leeds

Milne, J. S., Lonergan, M. E., Williamson, J., Moore, F. M. L., McMaster, R. and Percy, N. (1971). *Br. Med. J., 4*, 383

Milner, C. (1963). *Br. J. Psychiat., 109*, 294

Minor, A. H. and Ramirez, M. A. (1943). *Cancer Res., 2*, 509

Mirvish, S. S. (1971). *J. Natn. Cancer Inst., 46*, 1183

Mirvish, S. S., Cardesa, A., Wallcave, L. and Shubik, P. (1975). *J. Natn. Cancer Inst., 55*, 633

Mirvish, S. S., Wallcave, L., Eagen, M. and Shubik, P. (1972). *Science, 177*, 65

Mitchell, M. E. (1978). *Am. J. Clin. Nutr., 31*, 293

Mitra, M. L. (1970). *J. Am. Geriat. Soc., 18*, 67

Moore, M. R., Rohatgi, S. and Low, R. A. (1979). *Br. J. Obstet. Gynaecol., 84*, 293

Morgan, A. F., Gillum, H. L. and Williams, R. I. (1955). *J. Nutr., 55*, 431

Morgan, A. G., Kelleher, J., Walker, B. E. and Losowsky, M. S. (1976). *Gut, 17*, 113

Moriarty, M. J., Mulgrew, S., Malone, J. R. and O'Connor, M. K. (1977). *Ir. J. Med. Sci., 146*, 74

Morishige, F. and Murata, A. (1978). *J. Int. Acad. Prevent. Med., 5*, 1

Morley, G., Dawson, A. and Marks, V. (1968). *Proc. Ass. Clin. Biochem., 5*, 42

Mowat, A. P. (1968). *J. Endocrinol., 42*, 585

Murdock, D. S., Donaldson, M. L. and Gubler, C. J. (1974). *Am. J. Clin. Nutr., 27*, 696

Murphy, F. H. and Zelman, S. (1965). *J. Urol., 94*, 297

Myllyla, R., Kuutti-Savolainen, E. R. and Kivirikko, K. I. (1978). *Biochem. Biophys. Res. Commun., 83*, 441

Nambisan, B. and Kurup, P. A. (1975). *Atherosclerosis, 22*, 447

Nandi, B. K., Majumder, A. K., Subramanian, N. and Chatterjee, I. B. (1973). *J. Nutr., 103*, 1688

Narisawa, T., Wong, C. Q., Maronpot, R. R. and Weisburger, J. H. (1976). *Cancer Res., 36*, 505

National Food Survey Committee, Annual Reports (1950–80). Ministry of Agriculture, Fisheries and Food. HMSO, London

National Food Survey Committee (1973–81). *Trade and Ind., 10–38. British Business, 1–4.*

Neumann, C. G., Lawlor, G. J., Stiehm, E. R., Swendseid, M. E., Newton, C., Herbert, J., Ammann, A. J. and Jacob, M. (1975). *Am. J. Clin. Nutr., 28*, 89

Newmark, H. L., Scheiner, J., Marcus, M. and Prabhudesai, M. (1976). *Am. J. Clin. Nutr., 29*, 645

Nichol, C. A. and Welch, A. D. (1950). *Proc. Soc. Expt. Biol. Med., 74*, 52

Nicol, B. M. (1956). *Br. J. Nutr., 10*, 275

Nishikimi, M. (1975). *Biochem. Biophys. Res. Commun., 63*, 463

Nobile, S. (1974). *Med. J. Aust., 20*, 601

Norkus, E. P. and Rosso, P. (1975). *Ann. N.Y. Acad. Sci., 258*, 401

Odumosu, A. and Wilson, C. W. M. (1971). *Proc. Nutr. Soc., 30*, 81

—— (1973). *Br. J. Pharmacol., 48*, 326P

—— (1979). *Br. J. Pharmacol., 67*, 456P

Office of Population Censuses and Surveys (1970). Classification of Occupations. HMSO, London

O'Keane, M., Russell, R. I. and Goldberg, A. (1972). *J. Alcoholism, 7*, 6

Oliver, M. F., Heady, J. A. and Morris, J. N. (1980). *Lancet, 2*, 379

Olliver, M. (1967a). In *The Vitamins*, ed. Sebrell, W. H. and Harris, R. S., Vol. I, 2nd edn, p. 338. Academic Press, New York and London

—— (1967b). In *The Vitamins*, ed. Sebrell, W. H. and Harris, R. S., Vol. I, 2nd edn, p. 359. Academic Press, New York and London

—— (1967c). In *The Vitamins*, ed. Sebrell, W. H. and Harris, R. S., Vol. I, 2nd edn, p. 367. Academic Press, New York and London

Olusi, S. O., Ojutiku, O. O., Jessop, W. J. E. and Iboko, M. I. (1979). *Clinica Chim. Acta, 92*, 161

Omura, H., Tomita, Y., Nakamura, Y. and Murakami, H. (1974). *J. Fac. Agric. Kyushu Univ., 18*, 181

Orr, C. W. M. (1970). *Meth. Enzym., 18*, 59

O'Sullivan, D. J., Callaghan, N., Ferriss, J. B., Finucane, J. F. and Hegarty, M. (1968). *Ir. J. Med. Sci., 1*, 151

Paul, P. K. and Duttagupta, P. N. (1978). *Indian J. Exp. Biol., 16*, 18

Pauling, L. (1970). *Vitamin C and the Common Cold.* W. H. Freeman & Co, San Francisco

Pelletier, O. (1968). *Am. J. Clin. Nutr., 21*, 1259

—— (1975). *Ann. N.Y. Acad. Sci., 258*, 156

Pelner, L. (1944). *Ann. Allergy, 2*, 231

Peloux, Y., Nofre, C., Cier, A. and Colbert, I. (1962). *Annls. Inst. Pasteur, Paris, 102*, 6

Penney, J. R. and Zilva, S. S. (1946). *Biochem. J., 40*, 695

Pertoft, H., Back, O. and Lindahl-Keissling, K. (1968). *Expl. Cell Res., 50*, 355

Pijoan, M. and Lozner, E. I. (1944). *Bull. Johns Hopkins Hosp., 75*, 303

Pitt, B. and Pollitt, N. (1971). *Br. J. Psychiat., 118*, 237

Pitt, H. A. and Costrin, A. M. (1979). *J. Am. Med. Assoc., 241*, 908

Polgar, P. and Taylor, L. (1980). *Prostaglandins, 19*, 693

Portnoy, B. and Wilkinson, J. F. (1938). *Br. Med. J., 1*, 554

Poser, E. and Smith, L. H. (1972). *New Eng. J. Med., 287*, 412

Powels, T., Smith, I. E., Ford, H. T., Coombs, R. C., Jones, J. M. and Gazet, J. C. (1980). *Lancet, 1*, 580

Prasad, J. S. (1975). *Clinica Chim. Acta, 59*, 101

Price, J. M., Wear, J. B., Brown, R. R., Stalter, E. J. and Olson, C. (1960). *J. Urol., 83*, 376

Priest, R. E. and Bublitz, C. (1967). *Lab. Invest., 17*, 371

Prinz, W., Bortz, R., Bregin, B. and Hersch, M. (1977). *Int. J. Vitam. & Nutr. Res., 47*, 248

Pye, O. F., Taylor, C. M. and Fontanares, P. E. (1961). *J. Nutr., 73,* 236

Raineri, R. and Weisburger, J. H. (1975). *Ann. N.Y. Acad. Sci., 258,* 181

Ram, M. M. (1965). *Indian J. Med. Res., 53,* 891

Ramirez, I., Richie, E., Wang, Y-M. and van Eys, J. (1980). *J. Nutr., 110,* 2207

Ramirez, J. and Flowers, N. C. (1980). *Am. J. Clin. Nutr., 33,* 2079

Rao, N. V. and Adams, E. (1979). *Biochem. Biophys. Res. Comm., 86,* 654

Rebora, A., Dallegri, F. and Patrone, F. (1980). *Br. J. Derm., 102,* 49

Regnier, E. (1968). *Rev. Allergy, 22,* 835

Rikans, L. E., Smith, C. R. and Zannoni, V. G. (1978). *J. Pharmac. Exp. Ther., 204,* 702

Rinehart, J. F., Greenberg, L. D. and Christie, A. U. (1936). *Proc. Soc. Expt. Biol. Med., 35,* 350

Rivers, J. M. and Devine, M. M. (1975). *Ann. N.Y. Acad. Sci., 258,* 465

Roderuck, C., Burrill, L., Campbell, L. J., Brakke, B. E., Childs, M. T., Leverton, R., Chaloupka, M., Jebe, E. H. and Swanson, P. P. (1958). *J. Nutr., 66,* 15

Roe, J. H. (1954). *Meth. Biochem. Analysis, 1,* 115

—— (1967). In *The Vitamins,* ed. György, P. and Pearson, W. N., Vol. VII, p. 27. Academic Press, London, New York

Roe, J. H. and Kuether, C. A. (1943). *J. Biol. Chem., 147,* 399

Roeser, H. P., Halliday, J. W., Sizemore, D. J., Nikles, A. and Willgoss, D. (1980). *Br. J. Haemat., 45,* 459

Roitt, I. M. (1977). *Essential Immunology,* 3rd edn. Blackwell Scientific Publications, Oxford

Roos, D., van Schaik, M. L. J., Weening, R. S. and Wever, R. (1977). In *EMBO Workshop on Superoxide and Superoxide Dismutase,* ed. Michelson, A. M., McCord, J. M. and Fridovich, I., p. 307. Academic Press, New York

Rosenberg, H. R. (1945). *Chemistry and Physiology of the Vitamins,* p. 316. Interscience, New York and London

Rosenthal, G. (1971). *J. Am. Med. Assoc., 215,* 1671

Ross, R. and Benditt, E. P. (1964). *J. Cell Biology, 22,* 365

Rustia, M. (1975). *J. Natn. Cancer Inst., 55,* 1389

Ryan, W. L. and Coronel, D. M. (1969). *Am. J. Obstet. Gynec., 105,* 121

Samborskaya, E. P. and Ferdman, T. D. (1966). *Byull. Eksp. Biol. Med., 62,* 96

Sandler, J. A., Gallin, J. I. and Vaughan, M. (1975). *J. Cell Biol.*, *67*, 480

Sarji, K. E., Kleinfelder, J. and Brewington, P. (1979). *Thrombosis Res.*, *15*, 639

Sato, P. (1980). *Mol. Pharmacol.*, *18*, 326

Sato, P., Nishikimi, M. and Udenfriend, S. (1976). *Biochem. Biophys. Res. Commun.*, *71*, 293

Sato, P. and Udenfriend, S. (1978). *Archs. Biochem. Biophys.*, *187*, 158

Sauberlich, H. E. (1975). *Ann. N.Y. Acad. Sci.*, *258*, 438

Sauberlich, H. E., Dowdy, R. P. and Skala, J. H. (1973). *C.R.C. Crit. Rev. Clin. Lab. Sci.*, *4*, 227

Schaffert, R. R. and Kingsley, G. R. (1955). *J. Biol. Chem.*, *212*, 59

Schaus, R. (1957). *Am. J. Clin. Nutr.*, *5*, 39

Scheunert, A. (1949). *Int. Z. Vitam. Forsch.*, *20*, 374

Schlegel, J. U. (1975). *Ann. N.Y. Acad. Sci.*, *258*, 432

Schlegel, J. U., Pipkin, G. E., Nishimura, R. and Duke, G. A. (1969). *J. Urol.*, *101*, 317

Schlegel, J. U., Pipkin, G. E., Nishimura, R. and Shultz, G. N. (1970). *J. Urol.*, *103*, 155

Schorah, C. J. (1979). In *The Importance of Vitamins to Human Health*, ed. Taylor, T. G., p. 61. MTP Press Ltd, Lancaster

Schorah, C. J., Newill, A., Scott, D. L. and Morgan, D. B. (1979). *Lancet*, *1*, 403

Schorah, C. J., Smithells, R. W. and Scott, J. (1980). *Lancet*, *1*, 880

Schorah, C. J., Tormey, W. P., Brooks, G. H., Robertshaw, A. M., Young, G. A., Talukder, R. and Kelly, J. F. (1981). *Am. J. Clin. Nutr.*, *34*, 871

Schorah, C. J., Zemroch, P. J., Sheppard, S. and Smithells, R. W. (1978). *Br. J. Nutr.*, *39*, 139

Schrauzer, G. N. and Rhead, W. J. (1973). *Int. J. Vitam. & Nutr. Res.*, *43*, 201

Schropp, J. H. (1943). *Can. Med. Assoc. J.*, *49*, 515

Schwartz, A. R., Togo, Y., Hornick, R. B., Tominaga, S. and Gleckman, R. A. (1973). *J. Infect. Dis.*, *128*, 500

Schwartz, E. R. and Adamy, L. (1976). *Connect. Tissue Res.*, *4*, 211

Seyers, G., Sayers, M. A., Liang, T. Y. and Long, C. N. H. (1946). *Endocrinology*, *38*, 1

Shilotri, R. G. and Bhat, K. S. (1977). *Am. J. Clin. Nutr.*, *30*, 1077

Shukla, S. P. (1969). *Experientia*, *25*, 704

Siegel, B. V. (1975). *Nature*, *254*, 531

Siest, G., Appel, W., Blijenberg, G. B., Capolaghi, B., Galteau, N. M., Heusghem, C., Hjelm, M., Lauer, K. L., Le Perron, B., Loppinet, V., Love, C., Royer, R. J., Tognoni, C. and Wilding, P. (1978). *J. Clin. Chem. Clin. Biochem.*, *16*, 103

Sifri, M., Kratzer, F. H. and Norris, L. C. (1977). *J. Nutr.*, *107*, 1484

Sigell, L. T. and Flessa, H. C. (1970). *J. Am. Med. Assoc.*, *214*, 2035

Simonson, E. and Keys, A. (1961). *Circulation*, *24*, 1239

Skolnick, P. and Daly, J. W. (1977). In *Cyclic 3',5-Nucleotides. Mechanisms of Action*, ed. Cramer, H. and Schultz, J., p. 289. Wiley-Interscience Publications, London

Smith, A. D. M. (1961). *Lancet*, *1*, 1001

Smith, E. C., Skalski, R. J., Johnson, G. C. and Rossi, G. V. (1972). *J. Am. Med. Assoc.*, *221*, 1166

Smith, S. E. and Rawlins, M. (1974). *Eur. J. Clin. Pharmacol.*, *7*, 71

Smithells, R. W., Ankers, C., Carver, M. E., Lennon, D., Schorah, C. J. and Sheppard, S. (1977). *Br. J. Nutr.*, *38*, 497

Smithells, R. W., Sheppard, S. and Schorah, C. J. (1976). *Archs. Dis. Childh.*, *51*, 944

Smithells, R. W., Sheppard, S., Schorah, C. J., Seller, M. J., Nevin, N. C., Harris, R., Read, A. P. and Fielding, D. W. (1980). *Lancet*, *1*, 339

Sokoloff, B., Hori, M., Saelhof, C., McConnel, B. and Imai, T. (1967). *J. Nutr.*, *91*, 107

Sokoloff, B., Hori, M., Saelhof, C., Wrzolek, T. and Imai, T. (1966). *J. Am. Geriat. Soc.*, *14*, 1239

Sorensen, D., Devine, M. and River, J. (1974). *J. Nutr.*, *104*, 1041

Spector, R. (1977). *New Eng. J. Med.*, *296*, 1393

Spector, R. and Lorenzo, A. V. (1974). *Am. J. Physiol.*, *226*, 1468

Spencer, R. P., Purdy, S., Hoeldtke, R., Bow, T. M. and Markulls, M. A. (1963). *Gastroenterology*, *44*, 768

Spero, L. M. and Anderson, T. W. (1973). *Br. Med. J.*, *4*, 354

Spittle, C. (1971). *Lancet*, *2*, 1280

—— (1973). *Lancet*, *2*, 199

Srikantia, S. G., Mohanram, M. and Krishnaswamy, K. (1970). *Am. J. Clin. Nutr.*, *23*, 59

Stankova, L., Rigas, D. A., Keown, P. and Bigley, R. (1977). *J. Reticuloendothel. Soc.*, *21*, 97

Stein, H. B., Hasan, A. and Fox, I. H. (1976). *Ann. Intern. Med.*, *84*, 385

Stekel, A., Olivares, M., Lopez, I., Pizarro, F., Amar, M., Chadud, P. and Llaguno, S. (1980). *Pediat. Res.*, *14*, 74

Stephens, D. J. and Hawley, E. E. (1932). *J. Biol. Chem.*, *115*, 653

Stevenson, N. R. and Brush, M. K. (1969). *Am. J. Clin. Nutr.*, *22*, 318

Stewart, J. S. and Booth, C. C. (1964). *Clin. Sci.*, *27*, 15

Stokes, P. L., Melikian, V., Leeming, R. L., Portman-Graham, H., Blair, J. A. and Cooke, W. T. (1975). *Am. J. Clin. Nutr.*, *28*, 126

Stone, I. (1967). *Acta Genet. Med. Gemell.*, *16*, 52

—— (1972). *The Healing Factor 'Vitamin C' Against Disease.* Grosset and Dunlap, New York

—— (1980). *Med. Hypotheses, 6*, 309

Street, J. C. and Chadwick, R. W. (1975). *Ann. N.Y. Acad. Sci., 258*, 132

Streightoff, F., Bendor, B., Munsell, H. E., Orr, M. L., Ezekiel, S. R., Leonard, M. H., Richardson, M. E. and Koch, F. G. (1949). *J. Am. Diet. Assoc., 25*, 770

Subramanian, N. (1977). *Life Sci., 20*, 1479

Sulkin, N. M. and Sulkin, D. F. (1975). *Ann. N.Y. Acad. Sci., 258*, 317

Sviripa, E. B. (1971). *Zh. Nevropat. Psikhiat., 71*, 422

Szent-Györgi, A. (1928). *Biochem. J., 22*, 1387

Takiguchi, B., Furuyama, S. and Shimazono, N. (1966). *J. Vitam., 12*, 307

Taylor, G. (1966). *Lancet, 1*, 926

—— (1976). *Lancet, 1*, 247

Taylor, T. V., Rimmer, S., Day, B., Butcher, J. and Dymock, I. W. (1974). *Lancet, 2*, 544

Terroine, T. (1960). *Wld Rev. Nutr. Diet, 5*, 105

Thomas, T. N. and Zemp, J. W. (1977). *J. Neurochem., 28*, 663

Thomas, W. R. and Holt, P. G. (1978). *Clin. & Exp. Immunol., 32*, 370

Thornton, P. A. (1970). *J. Nutr., 100*, 1479

Tillmans, J., Hirsch, P. and Hirsch, W. (1932). *Z. Unters. Lebensmittel., 63*, 1

Tolbert, B. M., Chen, A. W., Bell, E. M. and Baker, E. M. (1967). *Am. J. Clin. Nutr., 20*, 250

Tolbert, L. C., Thomas, T. N., Middaugh, L. D. and Zemp, J. W. (1979). *Life Sci., 25*, 2189

Tonutti, E. (1937). *Z. Klin. Med., 132*, 443

—— (1938). *Klin. Wschr., 17*, 63

Trier, E. (1940). *C Vitaminstudier hos Syge og Sunde.* Munksgaard, Copenhagen

Tsutsumi, S., Nakai, K. and Nakamura, H. (1966). *Jap. J. Pharmacol., 16*, 443

Tuderman, L., Myllyla, R. and Kivirikko, K. I. (1977). *Eur. J. Biochem., 80*, 341

Turley, S. D., West, C. E. and Horton, B. J. (1976). *Atherosclerosis, 24*, 1

Ullrich, V. and Duppel, W. (1975). In *The Enzymes*, ed. Boyer, P. D., 3rd edn, Vol. XII, Part B, p. 253. Academic Press, London and New York

Vail, A. D. (1941). *J. Missouri St. Med. Ass., 38*, 110

Vallance, B. D. and Hume, R. (1979). *Br. Med. J., 1*, 955

Vallance, B. D., Hume, R. and Weyers, E. (1978). *Br. Heart J., 40*, 64

Vallance, S. (1977). *Br. Med. J., 2*, 437

—— (1979). *Br. J. Nutr., 41*, 409

Vanderkamp, H. (1966). *Int. J. Neuropsychiat., 2*, 204

Vann, L. S. (1965). *Clin. Chem., 11*, 979

Van Steirteghem, A. C., Robertson, E. A. and Young, D. S. (1978). *Clin. Chem., 24*, 54

Varley, H., Gowenlock, A. H. and Bell, M. (1976). *Practical Clinical Biochemistry*, Vol. 2, 5th edn, p. 249. William Heinemann, London

Veen-Baigent, M. J., Cate, A. R. T., Bright-See, E. and Rao, A. V. (1975). *Ann. N.Y. Acad. Sci., 258*, 339

Verlangieri, A. J. and Mumma, R. O. (1973). *Atherosclerosis, 17*, 37

Vilter, R. W. (1967). In *The Vitamins*, ed. Sebrell, W. H. and Harris, R. S., p. 457. Academic Press, New York and London

Vilter, R. W., Will, J. J., Wright, T. and Rullman, D. (1963). *Am. J. Clin. Nutr., 12*, 130

Vir, S. C. and Love, A. H. G. (1979). *Am. J. Clin. Nutr., 28*, 1934

Vobecky, J. S., Vobecky, J., Shapcott, D. and Munan, L. (1974). *Lancet, 1*, 630

Wada, F., Hirata, K., Nakao, K. and Sakamoto, Y. (1968). *J. Biochem. (Tokyo), 64*, 415

—— (1969). *J. Biochem. (Tokyo), 66*, 699

Waddington, J. L. and Crow, T. J. (1979). *Brain Research, 161*, 371

Waldo, A. L. and Zipf, R. E. (1955). *Cancer, 8*, 187

Walker, A. (1968). *Br. J. Derm., 80*, 625

Wapnick, A. A., Bothwell, T. H. and Seftel, H. (1970). *Br. J. Haemat., 19*, 271

White, A., Handler, P., Smith, E. L., Hill, R. L. and Lehman, I. R. (1978). *Principles of Biochemistry*, 6th edn, p. 1135. McGraw-Hill, Tokyo, London and New York

Willis, G. C. (1953). *Can. Med. Assoc. J., 69*, 17

Willis, G. C. and Fishman, S. (1955). *Can. Med. Assoc. J., 72*, 500

Wilson, C. W. M. (1975). *Ann. N.Y. Acad. Sci., 258*, 355

—— (1977). *Acta Vitam. Enzymologica, 31*, 35

Wilson, C. W. M. and Loh, H. S. (1973). *Lancet, 2*, 859

Wilson, J. and Langman, M. J. S. (1966). *Nature, 212*, 787

Wilson, T. S. (1972). *Geront. Clin., 14*, 17

Wilson, T. S., Datta, S. B., Murell, J. S. and Andrews, C. T. (1973). *Age & Ageing, 2*, 163

Windsor, A. C. W. and Williams, C. B. (1970). *Br. Med. J., 1*, 732

Winterfeldt, E. A., Eyring, E. J. and Vivian, V. M. (1970). *Lancet, 1*, 1347

Wokes, F. (1958). *Lancet, 2*, 526

Woodhill, J. M., Nobile, S., Silink, S. J. and Winston, J. M. (1974). *Aust. Paediat. J., 10*, 199

Woodruff, C. W. (1964). In *Nutrition*, ed. Beaton, G. H. and McHenry, E. W., Vol. II, p. 265. Academic Press, New York and London

Yamafuji, K., Nakamura, Y., Omura, H., Soeda, T. and Gyotoku, K. (1971). *Z. Krebsforsch., 76*, 1

Yeung, D. L. (1976). *Am. J. Clin. Nutr., 29*, 1216

Yew, M. S. (1973). *Proc. Natl. Acad. Sci., 70*, 969

—— (1975). *Ann. N.Y. Acad. Sci., 258*, 451

Yonemato, R. H., Chretien, P. B. and Fehniger, T. F. (1976). *Proc. Am. Ass. Cancer Res., 17*, 288

Young, E. G. (1964). In *Dietary Standards in Nutrition*, ed. Beaton, G. H. and McHenry, E. W., Vol. II, p. 299. Academic Press, New York

Zannoni, V. G. (1977). *Acta Vitam. Enzymologica, 31*, 17

Zannoni, V. G., Lynch, M., Goldstein, S. and Sato, P. H. (1974). *Biochem. Med., 11*, 41

Zannoni, V. G. and Sato, P. H. (1975). *Ann. N.Y. Acad. Sci., 258*, 119

—— (1976). *Fedn. Proc., 35*, 2464

Zloch, Z., Cerven, J. and Ginter, E. (1971). *Analyt. Biochem., 43*, 99

Zuskin, E., Lewis, A. J. and Bouhuys, A. (1973). *J. Allergy Clin. Immunol., 51*, 218

INDEX

abdominal cramps 118
absorption 13–15, 72
absorptivity 25
actinomycin D 19
adaptation 121
adrenal glands 15, 45, 57–8, 111
adverse effect *see* toxicity
age and ageing 55, 64, 66–8, 75, 124
alveolar bone 112
amines 45, 103, 104
amino acids 115–16, 117; *see also* individual amino acids
aminopyrine 103
3-amino-1,2,4-triazole 101
anaemia 38, 47, 53
arterial disease and atherosclerosis 52, 81, 95–100, 113–14, 124
ascorbate oxidase 24–5, 64
ascorbic acid-2-sulphate 17, 54, 116
assay 21–6, 46; *see also* measurement
asthma 53, 78, 111, 113

behaviour, disturbance 38, 45–6, 58, 86, 124
beneficial effects of vitamin C 93–114; *see also* hypovitaminosis C, scurvy
bile acids 50, 96
biosynthesis 11–13, 19, 102
bladder tumour 102
blood-brain barrier 18
blood vessels (microvaricosities, haemorrhage) 38, 43, 87–8, 124; *see also* arterial disease
body pool 16, 32–4
bone disease *see* skeletal disorders
brain 15, 45, 67, 87; amines in 45–6, 58
breast cancer 105, 107, 108
buffy layer *see* leucocytes
burns 77, 110, 118

calcitonin 107–8
calcium 120
cancer 55, 81, 100–7, 113, 122, 124

carbon dioxide 16, 17, 19, 80
cardiovascular disease 95–100; *see also* arterial disease
carnitine 34–5, 86, 124; biosynthesis 44
catabolic products 16–20, 126
cause and effect 85
cerebrovascular disease 99; *see also* arterial disease
chemotherapy 105
chlorpromazine 24
cholesterol 50–2, 95, 97–8; hydroxylation 50–1, 96; sulphation 54
chorea 46
cobalamin (vitamin B_{12}) 53, 119
collagen 34, 42, 52, 78, 98, 107, 109–12, 119–20, 124
colo-rectal tumour 102
common cold and respiratory infections 57, 76, 93–5, 113, 122–3
copper 44, 101, 119
coronary arterial disease *see* arterial disease
corticosteroids 19
cyanide 116
cyclic nucleotides 52–3, 55, 120
cysteine 21, 116
cytochrome P 450 *see* oxygenases

deficiency: vitamin C 42, 49–50, 58–9, *see also* hypovitaminosis C, reserves of vitamin C, scurvy; vitamins other than C 48, 87, 91–2, 125, 127
L-dehydroascorbic acid 11, 14, 17, 21, 37, 43, 77–8, 101; assay of vitamin C 21–6
deoxyribonucleic acid (DNA) 101
dextran 23; sedimentation of red cells 29
diabetes 55, 78
diarrhoea 118
2,6-dichlorophenol indophenol 21–4
dietary assessment 27–8; recall method 28

dietary vitamin C: adequacy 59,
124−5; and leucocyte 82−3, 91;
and plasma 82, 84, 91; influenced
by 35, 61, 64−9, 79, 125; prevent
hypovitaminosis C 91, 124;
prevent scurvy 81, 124;
recommended 66, 80, 91, 125,
assessment of 80−1; *see also*
food, megadoses, sources
2,3-diketogluonic acid 17, 22−3,
26, 36, 76, 101
dimethylamine 103; nitrosamine
103
dimethyl-thiazolyl-diphenyl-
tetrazolium bromide 24
2,4-dinitrophenylhydrazine 22−4,
26
disease: acute 30, 35, 55, 68, 75,
and C reserves 75−7; and
megadoses vitamin C 93−114;
chronic 35, 46, 55, 64, 67, 77,
and C reserves 77−9; *see also*
hypovitaminosis C, scurvy
diskinesia 46
distribution 14−16; *see also*
specific organ, tissue vitamin C
dopamin 44−6; and cyclic AMP
53; β-mono oxygenase 44−5
drug-metabolism 88, 118; enzymes
see oxygenases, P450-dependent
mixed-function; rate of 19, 48−
50, 80, 88, 116, 118

Ehlers-Danlos syndrome 42
Ehrlich ascites 101
elderly *see* age
epidermoid carcinoma 106
erythrocyte lysis 118
excretion 16−20, 32−3
expiratory flow-volume (EFV) 111
eye lens 15

familial polyposis 102
ferritin 53
fibrinolytic activity 99
ficoll (polysucrose) 23
folic acid and metabolites 44, 47,
53, 112, 125
food 66, 68; loss of vitamin C from
28, 64−6, 68; vitamin C content
64, 124−6; *see also* dietary
vitamin C
frankfurters 103
free radicals 56, 101

function of vitamin C 34−7, 38−60;
drug, cholesterol metabolism
48−52; immunity 54−7; other
roles 52−4, 57−60; reducing
agent 39−48

D-galactose 11
gingival inflammation 112
D-glucaric acid 19
glucose 11, 23−4, 78, 121−2
glucose oxidase 24, 121
glucose-6-phosphate dehydrogenase
118
glucuronide conjugation 116
glutathione 25, 39; dehydrogenase
25
gout 117
granulomatous disease 95
growth 89, 112, 115−16
guinea pigs 11−19 *passim*, 35, 44
47, 50, 80, 89, 97, 102, 111, 116,
121
L-gulonolactone oxidase 11−13
gut 13−15, 29, 77, 79, 117−18

haemoglobin 118
haemosiderosis 18, 19
half-life 16
health 89−90
heart burn 118
heart disease *see* cardiovascular
disease
heart muscle 15
hepatoxicity 103
histamine 111
homocysteine 22
3-hydroxyanthranilic acid 102
6-hydroxydopamin 45
hydroxylases 34, 40−5; lysyl 42−3;
prolyl 42−3; *see also* oxygenases
hydroxylysine 42
hydroxyproline 34, 42, 107−9, 120
hypercholesterolaemia 52, 98; *see
also* cholesterol
hyperlipidaemia 98
hypersensitivity 110−11
hypovitaminosis C 38, 96−7, 99−
100, 105, 124, 127; effect of
84−92, 97, behaviour 86, blood
vessels 87−8, drug metabolism
88−9, general health 89−90,
lassitude 86−7, wound healing
87; frequency 84−5, 90−1;
prevention 91, 124; vitamin C

levels in 74–5, 85, 90–1; *see also* scurvy

immunity   54, 93, 95, 113; and vitamin C 55–7, 122
infectious disease   93–5; *see also* disease, acute
infertility   120
institutionalisation   64, 68–70, 73, 75, 83, 85
interferon   57
iron   53
isoascorbate   42
isotopes of ascorbic acid   16, 19, 33, 35, 71–2, 79

2-keto-gulonolactone   13
kidneys   87; vitamin C in 15

lactation   78
lassitude   44, 58, 86–7, 124
leucocytes   15, 30–2, 46, 72, 93–4, 105, 108; vitamin C content 29–32, 35, 46, 107, and growth 89, and microvaricosities 88, effects on 64–80, 93, in drug metabolism 88, in hypovitaminosis C 74, 84–5, 94, in lassitude 86, in scurvy 74, 81, relation to diet 82–3, 91, relation to plasma 32, 61–3
leukaemia   105
liver   15, 19, 29, 48, 50, 96, 102–3; disease 77, 79, 88
lungs   15
lymphocytes   54–7; *see also* tissue vitamin C
lysine   34, 43, 109, 115

malignant disease   100–6; *see also* cancer
measurement of vitamin C: biological activity   34–7; choice of material 26–37; in plasma 28; in tissues 29–32; turnover and body pool 32–4; *see also* assay
megadoses of vitamin C   44, 52, 56–7, 60, 90, 127; dose 113–14, 122–3; possible toxicity 115–23; uses 93–114, cancer 100–7, cardiovascular disease 52, 95–100, common cold 76, 93–5, hypersensitivity 110–11, immunity 95, periodontal disease 111–12, skeletal disease 107–9, surgery

77, tissue healing 109–10, vitamin sparing effect 112–13
melanoma cells   101
metabolism of vitamin C: absorption 13–15, 72; biosynthesis 11–13, 19, 73, 102; body pool 16, 32–4, 63; excretion 16–20, 126; rate of 27, 34, 37, 46, 50, 61, 64, 69–74, 76–7, 79, 125
metal ions: and assay of vitamin C 21–2; and function of vitamin C 39, 41, 43–4, 101
metaphosphoric acid   26
N-methylamine   103
methylcholanthrene   102
N-methyl-N-nitroguanidine   104
methylurea   103, 104
mice   102, 120
monodehyroascorbic acid   11, 17
morpholine   103
mortality   90, 99, 115
mucopolysaccharides   43, 54, 98, 119
multivitamin supplements   92
muscle   15, 35–7, 67

1,2-naphthoquinone   22
nausea   118
neural tube defects   48, 92
neutrophils   54–7; *see also* tissue vitamin C
nitrites   103, 104
nitroso compounds   103–4
noradrenalin   44–6, 53, 124

oral contraceptives   19, 50, 71
oranges   124
osteogenesis imperfecta   108–9
oxalic acid   17–19, 117; *see also* catabolic products
oxygenases   40–52, 124; butyro-betaine 44; P450-dependent mixed-function 48–52; dopamine 44, 49; lysine 41–4; mixed function 19, 41, 48–52, 96, 118; proline 41–4

Paget's disease of bone   107, 108
periodontal disease   111–12
peroxide   13, 57, 101, 121
phenobarbital   19
phosphorus   120
physical performance   44
piperazine   103

pituitary gland 15
placebo trials 46, 85, 94, 99–100, 106, 110–12
plasma proteins 89
plasma vitamin C 15, 28–9, 32, 35, 45–6, 61, 70, 93; effects on 64–80; 93; in behavioural change 86; in hypovitaminosis C 75, 84–5, 91; in lassitude 86; in scurvy 75, 81; relation to diet 82, 84, 91; relation to leucocyte 32, 61–3
platelets 29, 54, 77; vitamin C *see* tissue vitamin C
pool size 16, 32–4, 36
population groups: at risk of hypovitaminosis C 74–5, 82, 85; at risk of scurvy 74–5, 81–2; vitamin C in 32, 37, 61–3, 73–5
potato 66, 104, 124
pregnancy 48, 55, 71, 73, 78, 120–1
pressure sore 110
procollagen polypeptide 34, 42
proline 34, 109, 111
prostaglandins 54
psychiatric diseases *see* behaviour, disturbance
puromycin 19

race and vitamin C 72–3
rats 45, 50, 57, 102, 112, 120
recommended intake *see* dietary vitamin C, recommended
rectal polyps 102
red cells 29, 118
redox indicators 21–4
redox potential 39, 40, 56
reducing agents 21–2; vitamin C as a 39–47
renal threshold 32–3
requirements for vitamin C: in disease 91, 93–114, 122–3, 125; in health 90–1, 114, 124–5; to prevent hypovitaminosis C 91, 124; to prevent scurvy 81, 124
reserves of vitamin C 26–7, 33, 38, 61–92; adequacy of 80–92, 94, 124; affected by 27, 61–80, age 66–8, class 65, disease 75–9, 93, 104, 110, institutionalisation 68–9, season 65–6, sex 69–71, smoking 71–2, race 72–3, *see also* population groups

salicylamide sulphate 116
sample preparation 26
sarcoma-180 101
schizophrenia 46, 86
scurvy 11, 16, 19, 32, 34, 38, 42–3, 46, 75, 97, 121, 124; cholesterol metabolism in 97; features 38, 43, 47, 82, 87; frequency 38, 82, 124; prevention 81, 124; vitamin C levels in 74–5, 81, 92; *see also* hypovitaminosis C
seasonal differences 98–9; in vitamin C status 65–6, 82, 99
sex differences in vitamin C status 69–71
skeletal disorders 43, 107–9, 119–20
smoking 71–2, 99
social class and vitamin C status 65, 71
sources of vitamin C 64, 66, 124–6; *see also* dietary vitamin C
spleen 15
stability of vitamin C 26
steroid hormones 57
sulphathiazole 110
sulphides 21
superoxide 41, 56–7
superoxide dismutase 56
surgery 77, 109

testes 15
thiamin 112–13, 125
thiocyanate 116
thiosulphites 21
thrombosis 99
thyroid 15
tissue healing 77, 87, 109–10
tissue vitamin C 15–16, 29–32; in leucocytes (buffy layer) *see* leucocytes; in lymphocytes 31; in neutrophils 31; in platelets 30–1, 35, 78; saturation 91, 94
toxicity 113, 115–23, 125
transketolase 113
transport of vitamin C 13–14, 45, 78
trichloroacetic acid 26
triglycerides 52, 98
trytophan 102
tumour 100–1, 103; *see also* cancer
turnover of vitamin C 16, 32–4
tyrosine 35, 58

uric acid   117
urine   34–5, 47, 107, 120; vitamin C
   in 32–3, 68, 76, 93, 110

vitamin C interference: blood and
   urine sugar   121; serum
   bilirubin 122; serum lactate
   dehydrogenase 122; serum
   transaminase 122; serum uric acid
   117, 122
vitamins other than C   112–13, 119;
   see also deficiency
vitamin-sparing effect   112–13
vitamin supplements   92; *see also*
   megadoses of vitamin C

warfarin   118
wound healing *see* tissue healing